THE CLINICAL LABORATORY MANUAL SERIES:

Immunohematology

Other Delmar titles in this Clinical Laboratory Manual Series include:

Dean/Whitlock: The Clinical Laboratory Manual Series: Clinical Chemistry
Flynn/Whitlock: The Clinical Laboratory Manual Series: Urinalysis
Hoeltke: The Clinical Laboratory Manual Series: Phlebotomy
Marshall: The Clinical Laboratory Manual Series: Microbiology
Russell: The Clinical Laboratory Manual Series: Hematology
Smith: The Clinical Laboratory Manual Series: Immunology

Also available from Delmar Publishers:

Davis: Phlebotomy: A Client-Based Approach
Fong/Lakomia: Microbiology for Health Careers, 5E
Hoeltke: The Complete Textbook of Phlebotomy
Marshall: Fundamental Skills for the Clinical Laboratory Professional
Walters/Estridge/Reynolds: Basic Medical Laboratory Techniques, 3E

THE CLINICAL LABORATORY MANUAL SERIES:

Immunohematology

Sheryl A. Whitlock, M.A., MT(ASCP) BB

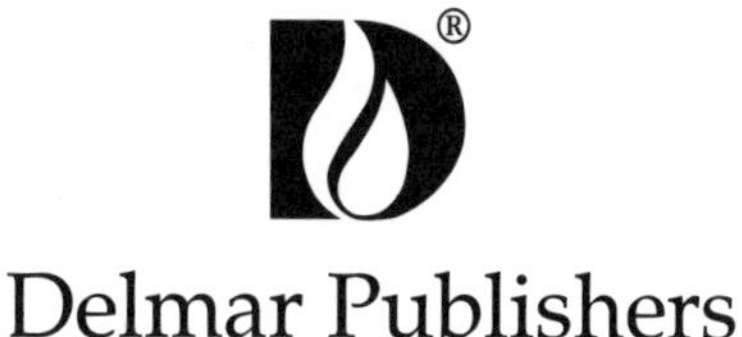

Delmar Publishers

an International Thomson Publishing company 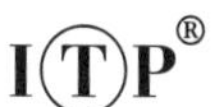

Albany • Bonn • Boston • Cincinnati • Detroit • London • Madrid
Melbourne • Mexico City • New York • Pacific Grove • Paris • San Francisco
Singapore • Tokyo • Toronto • Washington

Delmar Publishers' Online Services
To access Delmar on the World Wide Web, point your browser to:
http://www.delmar.com/delmar.html
To access through Gopher: gopher://gopher.delmar.com
(Delmar Online is part of "thomson.com", an Internet site with information on more than 30 publishers of the International Thomson Publishing organization.)
For information on our products and services:
email: info@delmar.com
or call 800-347-7707

Cover Design: joanne beckmann design

Delmar Staff
Publisher: Susan Simpfenderfer
Acquisitions Editor: Marion Waldman
Project Editor: William Trudell
Art and Design Coordinator: Rich Killar
Production Coordinator: John Mickelbank
Editorial Assistant: Sarah Holle
Marketing Manager: Darryl L. Caron

Printed in the United States of America

For more information, contact:

Delmar Publishers
3 Columbia Circle, Box 15015
Albany, New York 12212-5015

International Thomson Publishing Europe
Berkshire House 168-173
High Holborn
London, WC1V 7AA
England

Thomas Nelson Australia
102 Dodds Street
South Melbourne, 3205
Victoria Australia

Nelson Canada
1120 Birchmount Road
Scarborough, Ontario
Canada, M1K 5G4

International Thomson Editores
Campos Eliseos 385, Piso 7
Col Polanco
11560 Mexico D F Mexico

International Thomson Publishing GmbH
Konigswinterer Strasse 418
53227 Bonn
Germany

International Thomson Publishing Asia
221 Henderson Road
#05-10 Henderson Building
Singapore 0315

International Thomson Publishing–Japan
Hirakawacho Kyowa Builidng, 3F
2-2-1 Hirakawacho
Chiyoda-ku, Tokyo 102
Japan

2 3 4 5 6 7 8 9 10 XXX 02 01 00 99 98 97

Library of Congress Cataloging-in-Publication Data

Whitlock, Sheryl.
Immunohematology / Sheryl A. Whitlock.
p. cm.—(The clinical laboratory manual series)
Includes bibliographical references and index.
ISBN 0-8273-6867-4
1. Immunohematology—Laboratory manuals. I. Title. II. Series: Clinical laboratory manual series.
[DNLM: 1. Blood Grouping and Crossmatching—laboratory manuals. 2. Blood Groups—laboratory manuals. QY 25 W6131 1996]
RB45.W48 1996
612.1'1825—dc20
DNLM/DLC
for Library of Congress
96-28546
CIP

ACKNOWLEDGMENTS

Special thanks for their assistance in preparing this manual is extended to the following persons:

John C. Flynn, Jr., Ph.D
Montgomery County Community College
Blue Bell, Pennsylvania

Linda Pileggi
Montgomery County Community College
Blue Bell, Pennsylvania

CONTENTS

LIST OF LABORATORY EXERCISES

PREFACE

The *Clinical Laboratory Manual Series* is designed for use by instructors in vocational schools, community colleges, and the clinical laboratory environment. The purpose of the series is to give the medical laboratory technician the best education possible to meet the demands of the rapidly changing health care environment. Safety and quality control are strongly emphasized in all manuals.

This Immunohematology manual provides a hands-on approach to learning. Exercises are included throughout each manual to provide the learner with practice and feedback to enhance the learning experience.

Immunohematology is one of the four major departments in the clinical laboratory. This department, often known as blood bank, provides testing to ensure safe transfusion of blood and its components. Tests performed in the department include blood types, detection and identification of atypical antibodies, compatibility testing, and processing of donor blood and components. Education in the principles behind procedures is important to the success of the technician working in the laboratory. General test methods and the specific applications of these methods have been included in the manual. Results obtained in these tests are then applied to clinical conditions. In all laboratory departments, test results are important for diagnosis and treatment of clinical conditions.

The emphasis on safety is one feature of this manual. The student needs to adopt these safety practices as a part of the testing process. Universal Precautions have been outlined and included in all procedures with potential biohazard exposure. Clinical sites and laboratories will use practices similar to those incorporated in this manual as protection from accidental exposure to biohazardous materials. Quality control emphasis is also included in the text. This information provides the technician with an understanding of monitoring test practices to assure the clinician of accurate test results.

Each unit includes learning objectives, boldface terms found in a glossary, and review questions. As applicable, the units include information on specimen collection, test principles, specific test methods, evaluation of test results, and clinical conditions. Case studies are provided in some units so that the student may practice application of material included in the units. Often, the case studies will also emphasize application of material from other units when interpreting the test results. These case studies reflect the clinical conditions discussed in conjunction with testing protocol.

This manual is intended to serve as a compilation of information designed to provide the learner with an overview of blood bank test procedures. Additionally, common clinical conditions and how test results will be reflected in these clinical states is addressed. In summation, this manual is designed to provide information that will not only educate the learner, but also improve patient care.

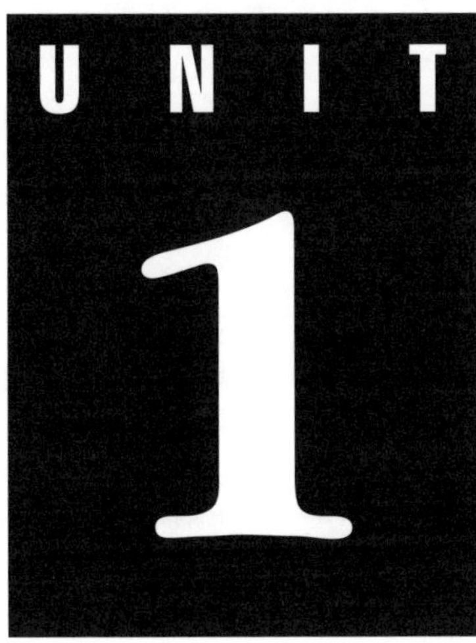

Introduction to Blood Bank

LEARNING OBJECTIVES

After studying this unit, it is the responsibility of the student to know the following objectives:

- Outline Universal Precautions guidelines.
- Discuss safety practices to avoid hand-to-mouth contamination.
- Describe disposal practices for biohazardous waste.
- List and discuss use of protective safety equipment for the blood bank laboratory.
- Briefly describe the criteria that would provide a quality specimen for analysis.
- Define all terms contained in the glossary.
- List tests performed in the blood bank laboratory.

GLOSSARY

anticoagulant substance that prevents the clotting of blood.

biohazardous having the ability to cause infections in humans.

blood bank major division in the hospital laboratory that performs blood type determinations, prepares and tests components for transfusion, and screens serum for atypical antibodies.

hemolysis destruction of red blood cells with release of the internal contents.

immunohematology study of blood-related antigens and antibodies as they may be applied to situations encountered in blood bank and transfusion service testing.

Universal Precautions set of guidelines developed to protect healthcare workers from exposure to infectious agents.

Wharton's jelly connective tissue substance coating the umbilical cord.

INTRODUCTION

This manual is designed to provide an introduction to basic test procedures in the blood bank. The **blood bank** is one of the major divisions of the clinical laboratory. It is the section of the laboratory that performs blood types, prepares and tests blood components for transfusion, and screens serum for atypical antibodies. The blood bank may be referred to as the "Transfusion Service" in some hospital laboratories. For the purposes of this manual, the term *blood bank* will be used consistently. Unit 1 outlines the tests performed in the department as well as safety measures for the protection of the technician. These safety practices will be applied throughout all procedures performed in this manual and in all areas of the clinical laboratory.

AN OVERVIEW OF BLOOD BANK TESTING

An understanding of the term **immunohematology** is necessary to prevent confusion on the part of the reader. Immunohematology refers to the study of blood-related antigens and antibodies as applied to situations encountered in blood bank or transfusion service testing. Immunohematology may not refer to the department located in the clinical laboratory. This department may be labeled Blood Bank or Transfusion Service.

Safety and quality control methods will be emphasized throughout the manual. Basic laboratory techniques are important for proper performance of blood bank tests and will be stressed as appropriate.

BLOOD BANK TESTS

The major test performed in blood bank and the most widely recognized in the general population is a blood type. The blood type detects antigens on the red cell surface. It includes an ABO group and an Rh type to provide a pair of notations (for example, A positive or B negative). Typing for additional antigens is performed as a special procedure and will be discussed in a later unit. Additional tests performed in the blood bank are covered in Table 1.1.

Many of the test methods have varying applications and are used in different conditions and situations. This will be emphasized and explained throughout the text.

SAFETY IN THE BLOOD BANK

The safety of workers in the laboratory is a major concern. There are categories of hazards that need to be addressed to ensure this safety. The categories applicable in the blood bank include biological, chemical, fire, mechanical, and electrical. The Occupational Safety and Health Administration (OSHA) defines the responsibilities of employers for providing safe environments for employees. It also requires the availability of written safety manuals for employees within the workplace.

Table 1.1. Some Tests Performed in the Blood Bank

- Antigen Testing
  ABO forwaard grouping
  Rh typing
- Antibody tests—performed on serum
  ABO reverse grouping
  Antibody screen
  Antibody identification
- Antibody tests—performed on cells
  Direct antiglobulin test
  Elution procedures
- Testing packed red blood cells and other blood components before transfusion
  Donor testing
  Pretransfusion testing with the patient's sample
  Follow-up testing of the donor and patient in a reported reaction to transfusion
- Testing for clinical conditions
  Hemolytic disease of the newborn (HDN)
  Hemolytic anemia

BIOLOGICAL HAZARDS

A primary focus of safety in the laboratory is **biohazardous** materials. All body fluids and tissues for analysis are considered biological hazards. A summary of substances posing potential biohazards is found in Table 1.2.

The Centers for Disease Control (CDC) publishes a set of safe practices referred to as **Universal Precautions.** This list of guidelines provides a basis for the protection of healthcare workers from biological hazards. OSHA requires that all healthcare workers comply with these guidelines when handling *any* sample or reagent that could pose a biohazard. Universal Precautions are outlined in Figure 1.1.

Of particular importance to laboratory workers is protection from needle puncture accidents. Needles should be discarded in puncture-proof containers labeled with the biohazard label (Figure 1.2). This method of disposal also applies for other items that are sharp or could contain sharp edges if broken, such as disposable test tubes and glass pipets.

When the precautions are followed, laboratory personnel are provided with protection from potential biological hazards. These procedures help prevent transmission of infectious agents such as hepatitis B virus (HBV) and the human immunodeficiency virus (HIV).

Laboratory workers should be aware that one of the major sources of biohazardous disease transmission is hand-to-mouth contact. For this reason, eating, drinking, and smoking in the laboratory are forbidden. An individual must be careful not to place inanimate objects or fingers into his/her mouth. Mouth pipet-

Table 1.2. Potentially Biohazardous Materials

- Whole blood samples
- Serum and plasma
- Urine
- Feces
- Other body fluids such as spinal or synovial fluid
- Reagents prepared from human blood products

Universal Precautions

- Consider **ALL** patients' blood and body fluids to be biohazardous regardless of diagnosis.
- Always wash hands before and after contact with patients.
- Wear gloves when handling blood, body fluids, tissues, or contaminated surfaces.
- Wear gloves and waterproof aprons, masks, and goggles if splashing can occur or during wound sterilization, endoscopy, dialysis, or postmortem procedures.
- Dispose of all needles in puncture-proof boxes, which must be accessible in all rooms.
- Minimize mouth-to-mouth transmission by keeping mouthpieces readily available on crash carts and in all areas where this need is possible.
- Clean blood and body fluid spills with a solution of bleach (10%) and water or with a hospital disinfectant.
- Immediately report all needle sticks, accidental splashes, and contamination of wounds by body fluids.

fig. 1.1. Universal Precautions recommendation.

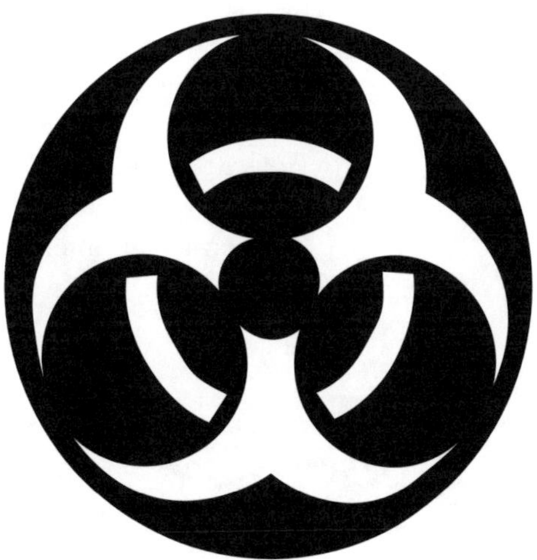

fig. 1.2. Biohazard label.

ting is strictly prohibited, and proper pipetting devices should be used at all times. Handwashing should be protocol after removing gloves and at all times before leaving the laboratory.

Barrier precautions are available and must be used by the laboratory worker as protection from potential biohazards. These barrier precautions include gloves, goggles, face shields, laboratory coats, aprons, gowns, and shoe covers.

EXERCISE 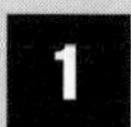 HANDWASHING TECHNIQUES

1. Turn on faucets and adjust water temperature using paper towels. This prevents contact with potentially contaminated faucets.
2. Wet the skin and apply the amount of soap indicated by the manufacturer.
3. Scrub hands vigorously in a circular motion for 3 minutes. Be careful not to touch any part of the sink.
4. Rinse and dry hands.
5. Turn off faucets with paper towel.

It is not necessary to wear all available protection at all times. The technicians should use judgment regarding the likelihood of exposure to aerosols, splashes, or skin contact. In addition, fluid-resistant laboratory coats and gowns provide additional protection from clothing and skin exposure to biohazards. The technician must also be prudent about changing gloves. Care must be taken to prevent contamination of inanimate objects and other persons.

Biohazardous waste must be discarded to render it no longer hazardous. Individual laboratories have methods for waste disposal. Waste is usually placed in containers labeled with a biohazard sign (see Figure 1.2). The waste is then autoclaved or incinerated. The option of using a disposal service is exercised by many institutions.

Accidental spills or contaminated surfaces must be wiped clean to render infectious agents ineffective. Biohazardous spills need to be decontaminated with a germicide such as 10% sodium hypochlorite (bleach) solution that has been proven to kill infectious agents. Daily cleaning of work surfaces with the same solutions may help prevent accidental contamination.

EXERCISE 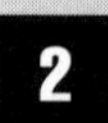 BIOHAZARD PROTECTION

Divide the class into groups and role play the following:

1. An instructor who is counseling a student who fails to wash his/her hands at the end of the laboratory session.
2. A student who notices another student placing a pencil in his/her mouth in the laboratory.
3. A laboratory supervisor who notices a staff member eating in the cafeteria while wearing an outermost lab coat.
4. A phlebotomist who notes that a fellow worker has discarded used gloves on the blood collection tray.

EXERCISE 3 REMOVAL OF SOILED GLOVES

The removal of soiled gloves must be done carefully to avoid contamination of skin. The following steps will prevent contamination. Wearing a clean pair of gloves, practice this procedure until you are comfortable with the steps.

1. With the thumb and index finger of one hand, pull the top of the glove on the opposite hand so that it is removed by turning it inside out. Be careful *not* to touch the skin on the wrist area above the top of the glove.
2. Place that glove into the palm of the still-gloved hand.
3. Using the hand with no glove, place the fingers of that hand inside the glove on the opposite hand.
4. Push the glove off so that it turns inside out and also covers the soiled glove being held in the palm.
5. The exposed surface is the inside of the second glove. Inside of that glove is the glove that was removed first and the soiled surface of the second glove.
6. Discard these soiled gloves into a biohazardous waste container.

Biohazardous reagents

Many of the reagents used for the testing of samples in the blood bank originate from humans. This applies both to antisera and cell products. Since these reagents are of human origin, they must be considered and handled as if they are biohazardous.

CHEMICAL HAZARDS

Chemicals may be hazardous with exposure. Hazards include toxicity, flammability, explosiveness, skin irritations, burns, or a combination of these. Chemicals are provided with a labeling system developed by the National Fire Protection

EXERCISE 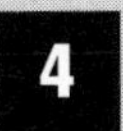 SAFETY PROCEDURE

Divide the class into small groups. The instructor will provide sample safety manuals. Each group will:

1. Review a safety manual.
2. Write a safety procedure for protecting the students from biohazards in the student laboratory.
3. Share these procedures.

Association (NFPA). Since chemicals are not a major component of the tests performed in the blood bank, they will not be considered at length here.

Employees need to be aware of the chemical hazards in the work environment. This is ensured by the OSHA requirement that material safety data sheets (MSDSs) be provided for each chemical by manufacturers and suppliers. These sheets must be available on site for the chemicals used in the laboratory area.

When reagent preparation is necessary, all containers should be labeled with the contents and concentration of the reagent. The expiration date, date of preparation, and name of the person who prepared the reagent should also be included.

Accidents can be reduced by using fume hoods, carriers for caustic chemicals, gloves, goggles, aprons, and other protective coverings when handling chemi-

EXERCISE 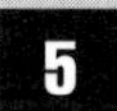

NFPA LABELS

The instructor will divide the class into small groups and provide samples of NFPA labels. Each group will:

1. Examine the NFPA labels on a minimum of five different chemical containers.
2. Determine how the sections of the label distinguish hazards.
3. Research the NFPA labeling system with materials provided by the instructor.
4. Determine if conclusions under #2 were correct.

EXERCISE 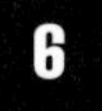

MSDS SHEETS

Instructors will divide the class into groups and provide each group with an MSDS sheet. The class will examine the sheet and determine the following:

1. The information provided on the sheet.
2. Possible adverse effects of the chemical. Some points to be considered may include:
   How should a spill of this chemical be handled?
   How should skin contact, inhalation, or other contact be handled?
   What specific barrier protection may be necessary with this chemical?

cals. Storage of volatile chemicals in specially ventilated cabinets is also necessary. As with biohazards, mouth pipetting is strictly prohibited to reduce the possibility of injury by exposure to caustic chemicals.

ADDITIONAL HAZARDS

Additional hazards in the blood bank include mechanical hazards encountered when working with equipment such as centrifuges and cell washers. Long hair should be tied back and loose clothing and jewelry secured or removed to prevent becoming entangled in moving parts.

Equipment and chemicals provide potential fire hazards. Fire extinguishers must be located throughout the laboratory. Technicians must distinguish the type of fire extinguishers (A, B, C) available and be experienced in their use. These are summarized in Table 1.3. Fire escape plans should be posted and fire drills conducted periodically.

Table 1.3. Fire Extinguishers.

Classes of Fire	Type of Extinguisher
A: Combustibles Paper Wood Cloth	A: Pressurized water A,B,C: Dry chemical
B: Flammable Liquids Grease Gasoline Oil	A,B,C: Dry chemical B,C: Carbon dioxide
C: Electrical	B,C: Carbon dioxide A,B,C: Dry chemical Halon

EXERCISE 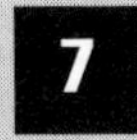 7 SAFETY EQUIPMENT LOCATION

The class should divide into small groups. Each group should:

1. Explore the student laboratory (or other area) and determine the location of all fire extinguishers.
2. Prepare a floor plan of the area to include location of:
   a. Fire extinguishers (labeled with type).
   b. Flammable chemical cabinets.
   c. Fire blankets.
   d. Safety showers.
   e. Exits.
3. Prepare a fire escape plan and include it on the floor plan.

SPECIMEN COLLECTION IN THE BLOOD BANK

PROCEDURES

All specimens for analysis should be collected by established procedures written in the laboratory specimen collection manual. The specimens must be properly collected, preserved, and identified. It is also necessary that the phlebotomist take care to collect a specimen that is free from **hemolysis.** The presence of free hemoglobin and cellular contents from lysis of red cells will interfere with the accuracy of results. This aspect of quality assurance helps to provide a specimen to obtain the most accurate results.

Most analyses in the blood bank are performed on clotted specimens. These specimens are collected by venipuncture or capillary puncture. The use of serum separator tubes is unacceptable. The silicone gel used in these tubes coats the red cells and interferes with the testing of those cells. Specific guidelines may be found in the laboratory specimen collection manual.

The use of anticoagulated specimens is unacceptable for most blood bank analyses. The binding of calcium by the anticoagulant adversely affects the activation of complement that is bound by some antibodies. The one exception is the direct antiglobulin test. A specimen collected in EDTA **anticoagulant** is acceptable for this procedure.

A blood sample may also be collected from the umbilical cord at birth. This sample is used to perform initial blood types and direct antiglobulin tests on the infant. Whereas the technician is not the individual responsible for collecting this sample, it is important that the technician be familiar with the correct collection technique. There is a connective tissue substance, known as **Wharton's jelly,** coating the cord. The specimen must be collected, avoiding contamination with this substance, by allowing blood from the cut cord to drip into the collection tubes. Labels are attached, and the sample is designated as a cord blood sample. The cord should not be "stripped" to force the blood to fill the tubes more quickly. This process is more likely to contaminate the sample.

LABELING

Individual specimens should be labeled at the time of collection with the information required by the institution. The minimum information is the patient's name, identification number, time and date of collection, and phlebotomist identification. Computer-generated labels are acceptable if applied at the time of collection and marked with the phlebotomist's initials.

STORAGE

Specimens are stored at 1° to 6°C for a minimum of 7 days. This is important for specimens that have been used for precompatibility testing. This will be discussed further in the unit covering compatibility testing.

MISCELLANEOUS SPECIMENS

Occasionally, the technician will be asked to evaluate amniotic fluid for the presence and titer of antibody. When this analysis is necessary, the technician should take great care to use the sample sparingly and freeze remaining fluid in small aliquots for later analysis. As always, fluids should be treated as biohazards and handled appropriately.

SUMMARY

The blood bank is a major department in the clinical laboratory. This department is responsible for providing transfusion components and evaluating clinical conditions related to antigen-antibody reactions as well as routine typings and screenings. Testing involves common tests such as blood typing and cross-matching prior to transfusion of blood components.

The proper collection and storage of specimens is vital to the performance of tests with accurate results. Proper specimen collection into tubes without anticoagulants is most often appropriate. Careful patient identification and labeling of the patient samples is established protocol.

Safety in all aspects of laboratory work is stressed. An employee in the blood bank must work in a manner to minimize accidents and exposure to biohazardous substances. The use of proper barrier protection and following Universal Precaution guidelines will prevent dangerous biohazard exposure.

Students are asked to consider the information presented in this unit as they progress through the following units. Safety and specimen collection will be emphasized throughout the manual and will become familiar themes as the manual is used on a regular basis.

REVIEW QUESTIONS

1. Barrier coverings are a category of items protecting the technician from biohazard exposure. Which of the following is not included in this category?
   a. sharps container
   b. latex gloves
   c. disposable aprons
   d. safety goggles
2. The Occupational Safety and Health Administration is for the
   a. disposal of laboratory waste
   b. protection of workers
   c. development of barrier protection
   d. accreditation of hospitals
3. Samples for blood bank tests are most often collected in
   a. citrated tubes
   b. red top tubes
   c. serum separator tubes
   d. heparinized tubes

4. Of the following, the test that is *not* performed in the blood bank is
   a. complete blood count
   b. blood type
   c. compatibility type
   d. screen for antibodies
5. Disposal of needles should take place in
   a. trash cans
   b. biohazard bags
   c. sharps containers
   d. all of the above
6. MSDS sheets provide information regarding
   a. AIDS exposure
   b. antigen contact
   c. chemical hazards
   d. air quality
7. Anticoagulated specimens may be acceptable for analysis of
   a. all blood bank analyses
   b. only pretransfusion screening
   c. direct antiglobulin testing
   d. antibody screen tests
8. When removing soiled gloves, the first glove removed is
   a. immediately discarded
   b. placed on any nearby surface
   c. held in the bare hand until the second has been removed
   d. placed into the palm of the still-gloved hand
9. Safety manuals must be made available in
   a. all laboratories
   b. areas in which biohazards are located
   c. hospital waiting rooms
   d. employee handbooks
10. Specimens tested in the blood bank should be labeled
    a. in the laboratory
    b. at the bedside
    c. at the time of testing
    d. while the blood is filling the tube

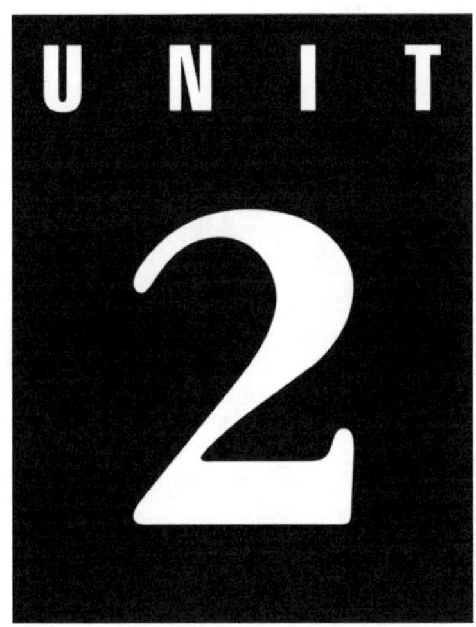

Basic Concepts of Immunohematology

LEARNING OBJECTIVES

After studying this unit, it is the responsibility of the student to know the following objectives:

- **Define the terms listed in the glossary.**
- **Discuss the components of coagulated and anticoagulated blood samples.**
- **Outline the structure and function of antigens and antibodies in the blood bank.**
- **Discuss antigens, antibodies, and complement and their relationships and reactions with each other.**
- **Outline the basic concepts of Mendelian genetics as they relate to antigen inheritance.**
- **Relate the concepts of antigens and antibodies to blood bank laboratory testing.**
- **Discuss the production and use of anti-human globulin reagents.**
- **Outline the theory of the anti-human globulin test.**

GLOSSARY

active immunization stimulation of antibody production by direct antigen contact.

agglutination clumping.

alloantibody antibody stimulated by exposure to exposure to a foreign antigen.

anamnestic response secondary antibody response.

antibodies proteins produced in response to stimulation by an antigen which then reacts with that antigen.

anticoagulant chemical substance that will prevent the clotting (coagulation) of blood.

antigenic ability to stimulate antibody production.

antigens biochemical substances that stimulate the production of an antibody.

anti-human globulin (AHG) sera reagent sera produced in a species other than human (usually a rabbit) that contains antibodies directed against human globulins; used to aid in the detection of antibody-coated cells in test procedures.

anti-human globulin (AHG) test test method that uses antibodies directed against human globulins to aid in detection of antibody-coated cells; used in specific tests in the blood bank.

atypical antibodies antibodies found either in the serum or on the cells that are unanticipated or not found under normal circumstances.

autoantibodies antibodies directed against antigens on an individual's red cells.

codominant genetic combination where both genes at a single loci are expressed.

Coombs' control cells (check cells) cells coated with an antibody used to confirm negative results obtained in indirect or direct antiglobulin tests.

Coombs' sera synonym for AHG sera.

decline phase phase of antibody production in which the level of detectable antibody is decreasing due to catabolism.

erythrocytes red blood cells.

foreign recognized as not belonging to a particular organism by the immune system of that organism.

hapten substance too small to stimulate antibody production without attaching to a larger molecule.

immune antibody antibody produced by direct stimulation with an antigen.

immunoglobulin synonym for an antibody.

in vitro outside of the body; in glass.

in vivo in the body.

indirect anti-human globulin test test method that promotes antibody attachment to cells *in vitro* and uses an anti-human globulin to bridge the antibody molecules on the cells; varied specific test applications.

lag phase first phase of immune response in which the levels of antibody are not detectable by testing.

leukocytes white blood cells.

log phase second phase of a immune response in which antibody production occurs in a logarithmic fashion.

natural antibody antibody produced without known exposure to the antigen.

passive antibody antibody administered to an individual.

plasma liquid portion of the blood; refers also to the liquid portion of a blood sample collected with an anticoagulant.

plateau phase response phase where antibody production is constant and detectable at stable levels.

polyspecific AHG anti-human globulin sera with multiple components; usually anti-IgG and anti-complement, but anti-IgM and IgA may be included.

primary response antibody response following initial antigen exposure.

prozone antibody excess that results in lack of agglutination.

rouleaux stacking of red cells like coins.

secondary response antibody response that follows any antigen exposure other than the first.

serum liquid portion of the blood after coagulation has occurred.

thrombocytes platelets.

titer concentration of antibody.

zeta potential net negative charge surrounding the surface of the red blood cell.

INTRODUCTION

The study of immunohematology merges aspects of areas of the clinical laboratory. The technician will be using specific technical information regarding blood groups and their characteristics as well as some basic aspects of hematology, immunology, and genetics. This unit will address some of the general topics that provide background for understanding and using the technical concepts of blood bank testing.

COMPONENTS OF BLOOD

Blood is the fluid providing the major transport system in the body. Blood is composed of cellular components suspended in a liquid portion called **plasma.** The plasma makes up approximately 55% of the blood volume and is composed of greater than 90% water. Proteins, nutrients, electrolytes, and other elements in transport are also contained in the plasma.

It is necessary to distinguish whether the liquid portion is plasma or **serum** when referring to a specific blood sample. Plasma is the fluid portion of a blood sample collected with an **anticoagulant,** such as EDTA (ethylenediamine tetraacetic acid) or sodium citrate. Serum, on the other hand, is the fluid portion of a blood sample that has clotted. Serum is the liquid blood component most often used in blood bank testing.

The cellular components suspended in the plasma are summarized in Table 2.1. These cellular components have different functions. The **erythrocyte** is the major cellular component considered in this manual. **Leukocytes** and **thrombocytes** will be considered briefly in this text.

FUNCTION OF BLOOD

The blood performs a variety of functions in the body. The main function is the transport of oxygen to the tissues and carbon dioxide to the lungs for expiration. It is the erythrocytes that perform this function. Blood bank testing uses erythrocytes and serum or plasma. These red blood cells carry antigens on their cell surface that are detected in testing. The plasma or fluid portion of the blood carries antibodies that are also detected and identified in serum tests in the blood bank. Additional functions of the blood are summarized in Table 2.2.

A final important function of blood is coagulation. Coagulation protects the body by preventing bleeding. This function is noteworthy in blood bank testing for two reasons. First, clotted samples are used for most blood bank testing. In

Table 2.1. Cellular Components of the Blood

Erythrocytes (red blood cells)
Leukocytes (white blood cells)
Thrombocytes (platelets)

EXERCISE 8 DISTINGUISHING PLASMA FROM SERUM

Students should work in pairs. All students should wear gloves and protective eyewear. In addition, safety precautions for needle disposal and safe centrifugation should be followed.

1. Each pair of students performs a venipuncture with one student serving as the phlebotomist and the second student serving as the patient.
2. A lavender top (EDTA) and a red-top nonanticoagulated specimen should be collected from each student.
3. Sufficient time is allowed for the red-top specimen to clot.
4. The tubes are centrifuged. Operation of the centrifuge should follow manufacturer's instructions.
5. Wearing gloves, each tube is examined to distinguish clot formation in the red-top specimen from the total liquid state of the EDTA specimen.
6. Repeat centrifugation, if necessary.
7. Specimens are separated, and the serum and plasma are labeled.
8. Each pair should have their work evaluated by the instructor.
9. Specimens may be saved for future exercises, if appropriate.
10. All biohazardous materials should be discarded in a puncture-proof biohazard container.

addition, when transfusion of blood components is considered, replacement of deficient coagulation factors may be necessary.

IMMUNOLOGICAL PRINCIPLES

The primary immunological components are **antigens** and **antibodies.** These components provide the basis for blood bank testing and reactions. There is a cardinal rule for antigens and antibodies as they relate to the blood bank. This rule is that antigens are found on red blood cells and antibodies are found in the serum or plasma. There are some exceptions to this rule. These exceptions will be noted, as necessary, in this manual.

Table 2.2. Functions of Blood

- Transport of nutrients, hormones, and chemical substances to the tissues
- Transport of waste products to site of removal
- Respiration: transporting oxygen to the tissues and carbon dioxide to the lungs
- Immunological protection by white cells
- Coagulation of the blood
- Phagocytosis of waste materials

ANTIGENS

Antigen Characteristics

Antigens are substances that have the capability to stimulate the production of an antibody. The chemical nature of antigens can be protein, carbohydrate, lipopolysaccharide, or nucleic acid. In order to stimulate antibody production, the substance must have a molecular weight of greater than 10,000. The larger the molecular weight, the more likely the substance will stimulate the production of an antibody. Small substances known as **haptens** must be bound to a larger substance to provide sufficient molecular weight to stimulate the production of antibody.

Complexity and stability are important for a substance to act as an antigen. The more complex the molecule, the more likely the substance will serve as an antigen. A molecule that is unstable and likely to degrade is less likely to stimulate an antibody response.

Another primary factor for a substance to be **antigenic** within the body is that the substance be **foreign**. A substance recognized by the body as "self" will not stimulate an antibody response in that person. Foreign antigens originate outside of the body.

Antigen Location

Antigens are located throughout the human body. The antigens present are determined by inheritance. Antigens are found on cells, on tissue surfaces, and in plasma and other body fluids. For the most part, antigens in blood bank testing are found on the surface of the red cells.

The physical location of the antigen on the red cell membrane varies, depending on the specific antigen. Some antigens protrude from the surface, whereas others are an integral part of the cell membrane.

ANTIBODIES

Antibody Characteristics

An antibody is a protein. It is produced in response to stimulation with an antigen. The antibody produced is specific for the stimulating antigen and will react with that antigen. An antibody molecule is also called an **immunoglobulin**.

EXERCISE 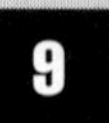 ANTIGEN EXPOSURE

The student should evaluate each of the situations below and determine the source of the antigen that would stimulate the formation of an antibody:

1. A measles immunization.
2. Hayfever.
3. A bee sting.
4. A blood transfusion.

The monomeric immunoglobulin molecule consists of four amino acid chains attached by disulfide bonds. The molecule is a Y shape with a hinge area. The chains consist of two heavy chains and two light chains (Figure 2.1). These chains are held together by disulfide bonds. Each of the four chains has two areas. The areas are labeled a constant portion and a variable portion (Figure 2.1).

Immunoglobulin molecules are composed of three fragments linked together by the hinge area. When immunoglobulin molecules are cleaved by enzymes, three distinct fragments are produced. The fragments are two (2) antigen binding fragments, FAB, and one (1) crystallizable fragment, FC, for each monomeric immunoglobulin unit (see Figure 2.1). The FAB portions bind the specific antigen during antigen-antibody reactions. The FC portion has numerous functions including placental attachment, complement binding, and macrophage binding.

Monomeric units may be combined. These polymeric units may be dimers (two units), trimers (three units), or pentamers (five units). These polymeric units have a higher molecular weight.

Immunoglobulin Classes

Five distinct classes of immunoglobulins are known. These are designated IgG, IgM, IgA, IgD, and IgE. For defining characteristics of these classes, see Table 2.3. Antibodies detected in the blood bank are primarily IgG and IgM. IgG is a monomer, whereas IgM is a pentamer. This structure difference makes IgM a much larger molecule (see Figure 2.2).

Antibody Production

Antibodies are produced by B lymphocytes. When first exposed to an antigen, lymphocytes are stimulated by that antigen. The lymphocytes process the antigen. Some lymphocytes are transformed into plasma cells and some into mem-

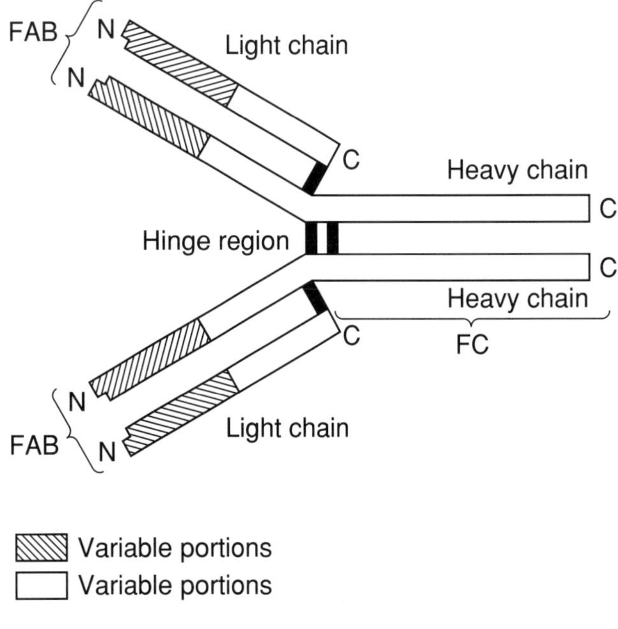

fig. 2.1. Labeled immunoglobulin monomer.

Table 2.3. Characteristics of Immunoglobulin Molecules

Characteristic	IgM	IgG	IgA	IgE	IgD
Molecular weight	900,000	160,000	360,000	200,000	160,000
Sedimentation coefficient	19S	7S	11S	8S	7S
Structure	Pentamer	Monomer	Dimer	Monomer	Monomer
Half-life (days)	5	21	6	2	3

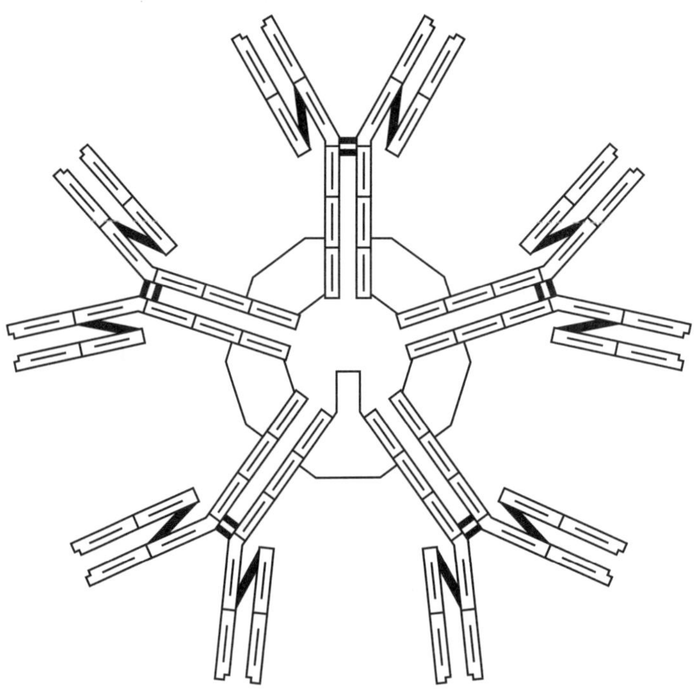

IgM immunoglobulin

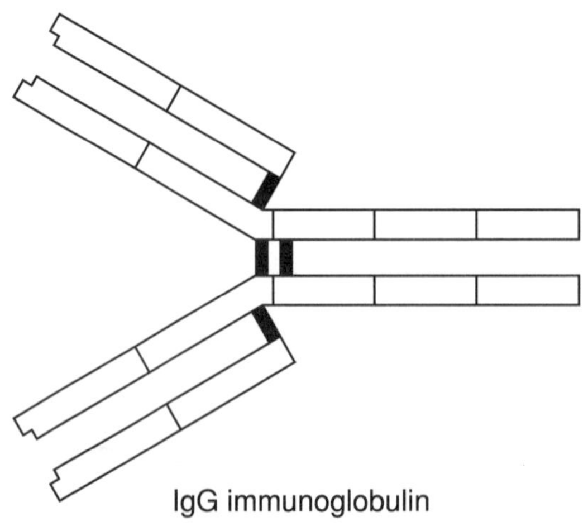

IgG immunoglobulin

fig. 2.2. Comparison of IgM pentamer and IgG monomer.

ory cells. These plasma cells produce an antibody specific for the stimulating antigen. Memory cells are stored and will transform and produce the specific antibody at any time the body is challenged with the antigen.

Antibody production begins upon antigen exposure. This initial exposure starts the **primary response**. During the primary response, the antibody production starts slowly with a **lag phase** (see Figure 2.3). During this lag, no antibody is detectable in testing because the antibody concentration is very low.

The **log phase** follows the lag phase. It represents a period of time when the antibody is produced in a logarithmic fashion (see Figure 2.3). During this phase, the IgM antibody rises first, followed by the IgG.

The third phase of the primary response is the **plateau phase,** where the antibody production remains stable. This is followed by the final **decline phase.** During this time, antibody is being catabolized and the detectable level of antibody is decreasing.

A subsequent exposure results in a **secondary** or **anamnestic response** (see Figure 2.3). This response differs from the primary response in several ways. With regard to time, a secondary response has a shorter lag phase and a longer plateau and the antibody titer stays higher much longer, providing it with a longer decline phase. The antibody produced in the secondary phase differs. In this secondary phase, IgG, not IgM, antibodies are the primary antibody class produced. Finally, the levels of antibody **(titer)** rise higher than those in a primary response. This increase may be as much as tenfold.

TERMINOLOGY

When antibodies are stimulated by direct contact with the antigen, it is known as **active immunization**. These antibodies are **immune antibodies**. Active immunization occurs in transfusion or pregnancy. Throughout this manual, immune antibodies will be discussed and referred to as **atypical antibodies**. These atypical antibodies will appear in the patient's serum and could result in a clinical situation such as hemolytic disease of the newborn (HDN) or hemolytic transfusion reaction (HTR).

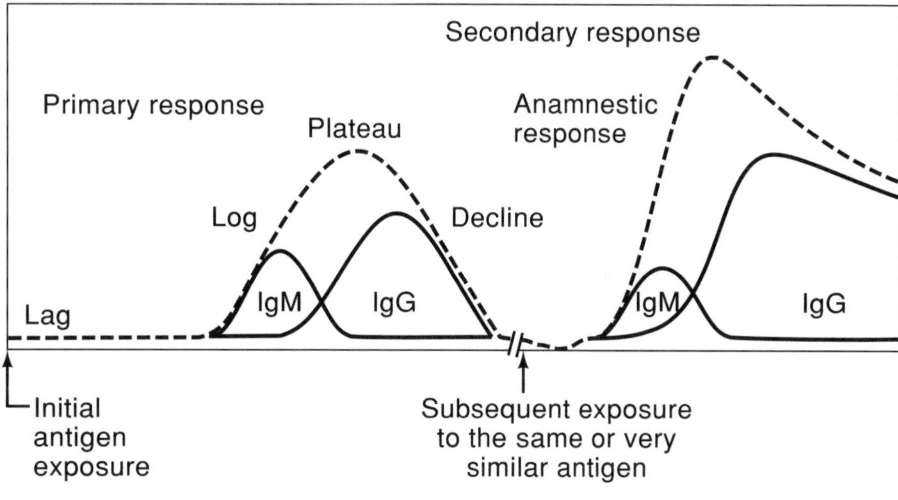

fig. 2.3. Primary and secondary immune response.

In contrast, antibody formation may occur without apparent antigen exposure. There is an antigen responsible for stimulating production of the antibodies, but its exact nature is not known. These antibodies are known as **natural antibodies**. Natural antibodies are found primarily in the ABO blood group system.

Antibodies may also be helpful in counteracting antigen exposure. These antibodies are usually administered by injection. These are termed **passive antibodies**. Examples include Rh immune globulin, used to prevent hemolytic disease of the newborn, and hepatitis B immune globulin, which counteracts exposure to the hepatitis B virus.

Antibodies produced in response to foreign antigens are designated **alloantibodies**. This is contrasted to **autoantibodies** formed in response to antigens on the cells of the individual. Autoantibodies are found in clinical conditions such as autoimmune hemolytic anemia (AIHA).

ANTIGEN-ANTIBODY REACTIONS

Once an antibody is produced, it has the capability to react with its specific antigen. This specificity provides the basis for most blood bank tests. Factors influencing antigen-antibody reactions are summarized in Table 2.4.

The factors summarized in Table 2.4 combine to influence antigen-antibody reactions. Visualization of reactions may be by **agglutination**, hemagglutination, precipitation, flocculation, or hemolysis. Antigen-antibody reactions in blood bank tests are visualized by hemagglutination and or hemolysis.

AGGLUTINATION

Agglutination of red blood cells (hemagglutination) and hemolysis are two methods to visualize antigen-antibody reactions in blood bank tests. Agglutination differs from precipitation. In a precipitation reaction, the antigen is one that is soluble in the reacting solution. When this soluble antigen combines with the antibody, the complex cross links to other complexes and forms small particles that "precipitate" or fall out of the solution. This makes the reaction visible.

Agglutination involves an antigen that is a particle or is attached to a particle (such as a red blood cell). Agglutination occurs in two stages. When the antibody

Table 2.4. Factors Which Influence Antigen-Antibody Reactions

- Specificity—each antibody is specific for the antigen that stimulated its production.
- Bonding—noncovalent bonds are involved in the attachment of antigens to antibodies.
- Physical "fit"—the fit of the antigen and antibody depend on compatible shapes that allow the antigen and antibody to attach with strong bonds. This is called a lock and key mechanism.
- Concentration of antigen and antibody—both antigens and antibodies must be present in optimal concentrations; excess antibody will result in a situation known as **prozone** phenomenon.
- Temperature—optimal temperature of reactivity for a specific antibody will expedite the combination of antigen and antibody.
- Time—incubation time must be that which is optimal for the specific antibody. General guidelines are a range of 15 to 60 minutes for optimal antigen-antibody attachment.
- pH—a pH of 7.0 is maintained for most antigen-antibody reactions.
- Surface charge—a net negative charge known as zeta potential surrounds the red cells. The reduction of this charge influences the ability of antigen and antibody to combine.

EXERCISE 10 PROZONE PHENOMENON

In small groups using the research material provided by the instructor:

1. Research the concept of prozone phenomenon.
2. Determine its effect on antigen-antibody reactions.
3. Write a paragraph summarizing this information.
4. Share with the class.

EXERCISE 11 OPTIMUM TEMPERATURE OF REACTIVITY

Using research materials provided by the instructor, each student should:

1. Research the optimum temperature for ABO and Rh blood group antibodies.
2. Prepare a chart summarizing this information.
3. Hand in work to instructor to check correctness of information.

attaches to an antigen on one cell, the free arm of the immunoglobulin monomer is free to attach to an antigen on a second red cell. This creates a crosslink. Multiple crosslinks create a lattice visualized as agglutination (see Figure 2.4).

The first stage of agglutination is sensitization, or the attachment of antibody to the antigen molecules. The second stage is lattice formation, or agglutination. This lattice formation creates the visible reaction. During lattice formation, the cross-linking of the cells is affected most by **zeta potential** (see Figure 2.5). This net negative charge surrounding the cells causes them to repel one another. It affects the ability of those cells to come close enough for lattice formation to occur. Reduction of zeta potential aids lattice formation. Some methods of zeta potential reduction include suspension of the cells in isotonic saline, addition of a substance, such as albumin, LISS (low ionic strength saline), PEG (polyethylene glycol), or anti-human globulin reagent, or treatment of the cells with enzymes.

GRADING AGGLUTINATION REACTIONS

When the process of agglutination has occurred in the test tube, it is necessary to determine the strength of the reaction. The reaction mixture of cells and serum (or antisera) is spun in a serological centrifuge for the appropriate amount of time. A serological centrifuge is represented in Figure 2.6. When the centrifuging is complete, the cells appear as a compressed cell button in the bottom of the tube. Surrounding this button is the remaining serum or antisera.

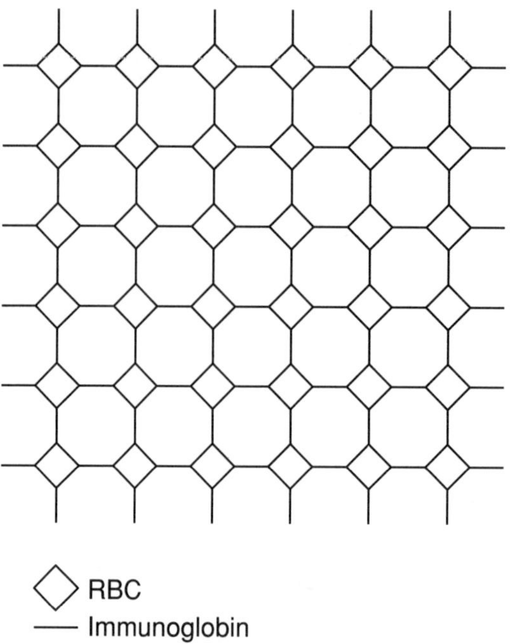

fig. 2.4. Lattice formation stage of antigen-antibody attachment.

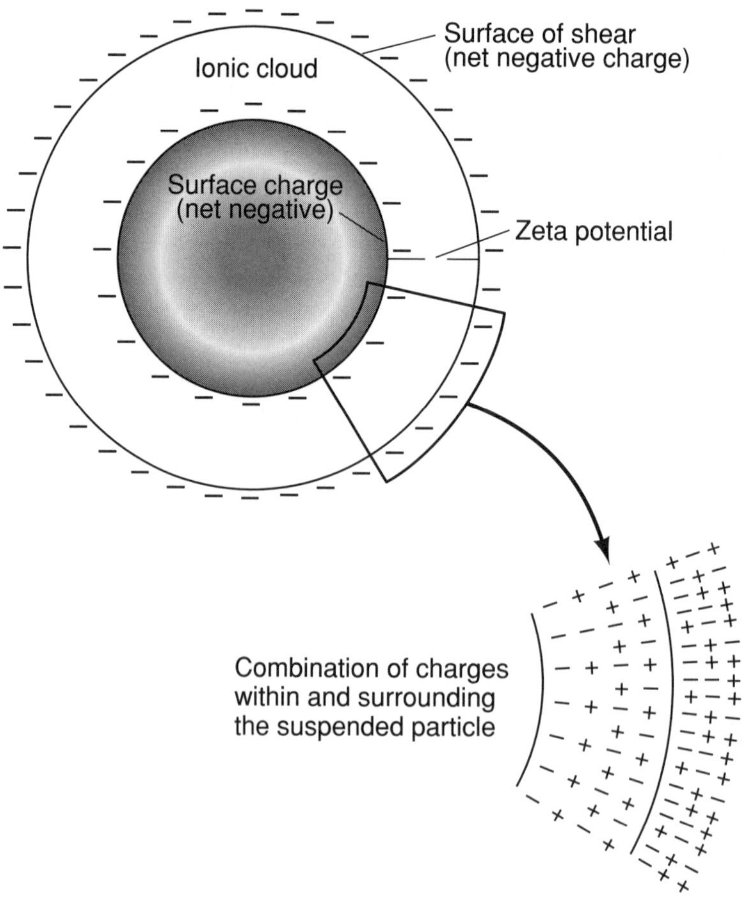

fig. 2.5. Zeta potential.

Each tube is first observed for hemolysis by examining the supernatant fluid for red or pink color. Hemolysis is noted and considered a positive reaction if it is present.

To examine the reactants for agglutination, good lighting is used, preferably with a magnification mirror. Figure 2.7 shows an agglutination viewer that may be used for this purpose. Each tube is gently shaken, and the cell button is observed as it becomes detached from the bottom of the tube. As the button becomes dislodged, the tube is tilted and the reflection of the fluid is examined in the mirror as it flows up the side of the tube. The technician examines the fluid for agglutinates or clumps of red cells. The button is also observed during the tilt-

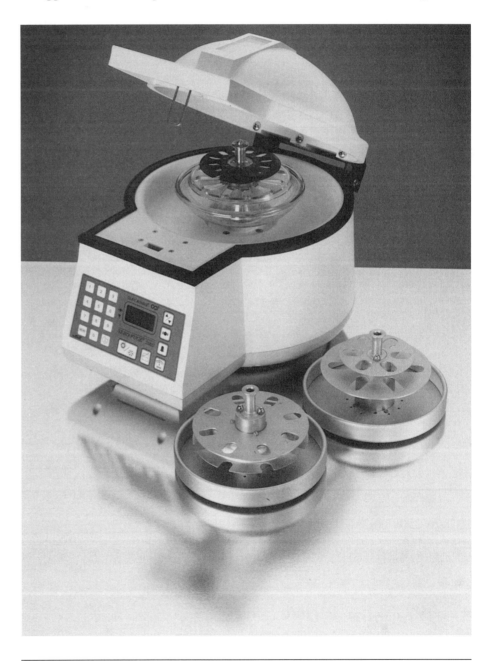

fig. 2.6. Serological centrifuge. (Courtesy of Becton Dickinson Primary Care Diagnostics; Clay Adams and SEROFUGE are trademarks of Becton Dickinson and Company.)

ing process. The technician notes whether the button is becoming dislodged in clumps or swirling as the cells break free. The final determination of agglutination strength is determined at the point where the entire cell button is dislodged from the bottom of the tube.

The grading of agglutination takes place at this point in the procedure. This grading is done by a standard system, with results ranging from a negative reaction graded as a 0 (zero) to a complete agglutination reaction, graded as 4+ (four plus) (see Figure 2.8). The grading scheme and the criteria for making a determination of the final grade of the reaction are outlined in Table 2.5. When recording the grading for each tube on a worksheet, a negative reaction must be recorded as a 0 (zero), never as a negative mark (−). Negative marks may be readily transformed to positive marks. Since worksheets are legal documents that may be used in court cases, the use of the negative sign is unacceptable. The positive reactions are recorded using either a number followed by a plus (+) sign or hash marks (see Table 2.5).

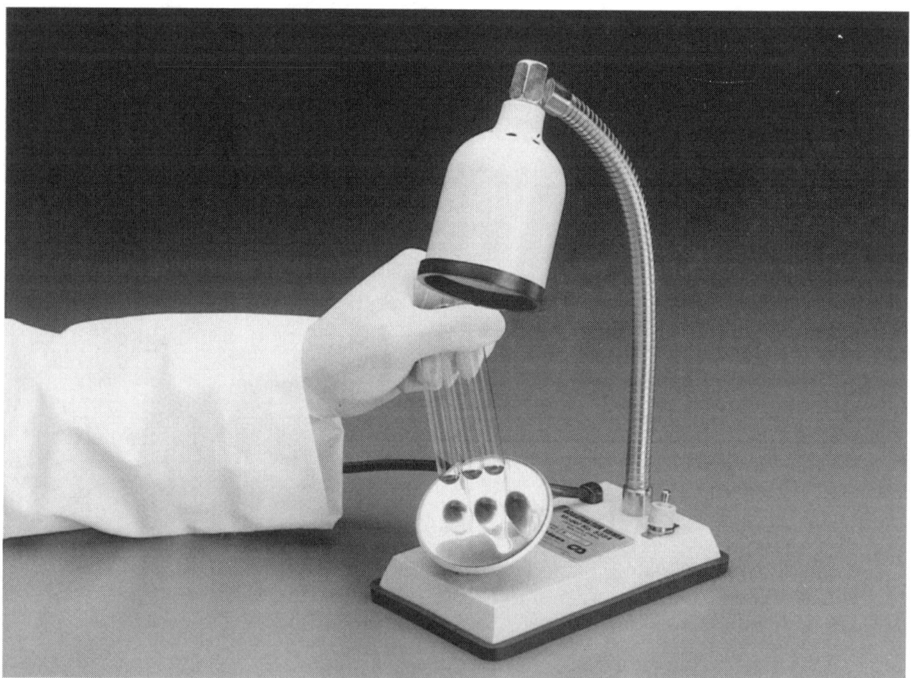

fig. 2.7. Agglutination viewer with magnifying mirror. (Courtesy of Becton Dickinson Primary Care Diagnostics; Clay Adams and SEROFUGE are trademarks of Becton Dickinson and Company.)

Table 2.5. Grading of Agglutination

Grade	Description
Negative	No clumps or aggregates
Weak (±)	Tiny clumps or aggregates barely visible macroscopically or to the naked eye
1+	A few small aggregates visible macroscopically; background supernatant cloudy
2+	Medium size aggregates; clear background
3+	Several large aggregates; clear background
4+	One solid aggregate; clear supernatant

Reaction Grading

The degree of red cell agglutination observed in any blood bank test procedure is significant and should be recorded. A system of grading is illustrated.

	Description	Reaction*	Grade
a.	Button breaks into two or three clumps after being dislodged. Background is clear.	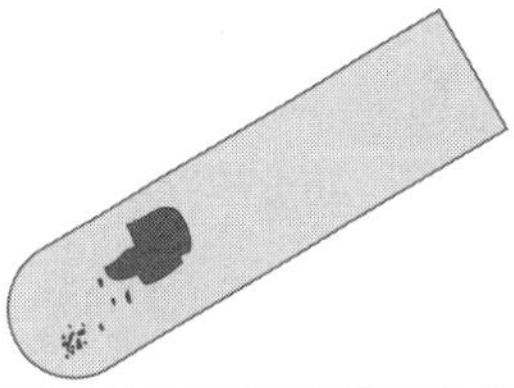	++++ 4+
b.	Button breaks into four to six large clumps. Background is clear.	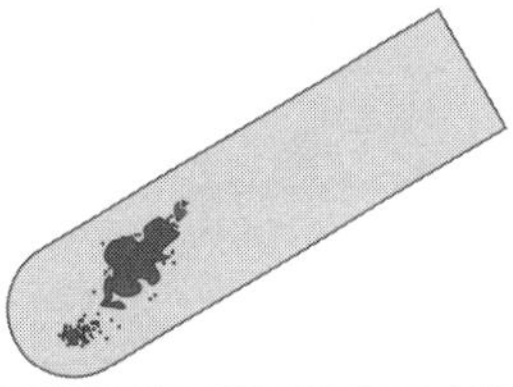	+++ 3+
c.	Button breaks into many small clumps. Background remains clear.	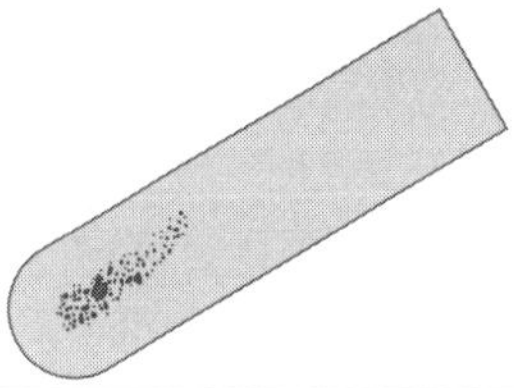	++ 2+
d.	Button breaks into numerous tiny clumps. Background becomes cloudy.	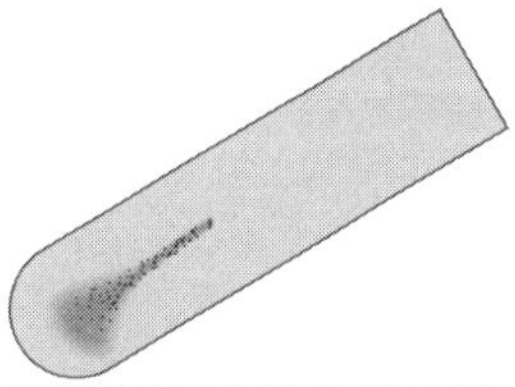	+ 1+
e.	Very fine agglutinates in a sea of free cells.	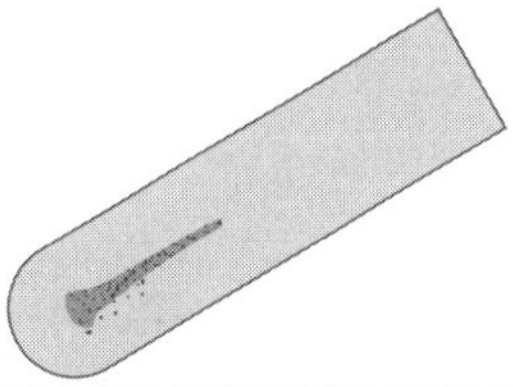	+w +w
f.	No visible agglutinates.	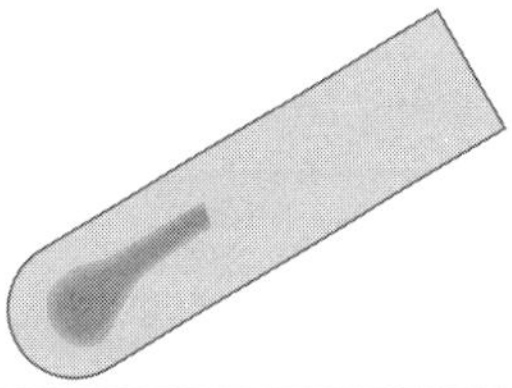	0 Neg.

fig. 2.8. Agglutination grading. a. 4+; b. 3+; c. 2+; d. 1+; e. +weak; f. negative.

EXERCISE 12 GRADING AGGLUTINATION REACTIONS

In small groups, the students should do the following:

1. Wearing gloves and protective eyewear, examine samples of agglutination provided by the instructor.
2. Examine the liquid of each tube for hemolysis. When doing this, the student is examining the supernatant liquid for the presence of a red or pink color. If the supernatant does not have this color, the result is negative. If the color is present, the result is positive. This examination may take place against a white background.
3. Each tube is examined for agglutination using an agglutination viewer with a magnifying mirror.
4. The tube is shaken gently and tilted so that the supernatant flows up the side of the tube.
5. Looking into the agglutination mirror, the student looks at the button and at the supernatant liquid as it moves up the side of the tube. Clumps of cells will indicate a positive reaction.
6. No determination of a positive reaction is made until the *entire button* has become dislodged from the bottom.
7. When the button is dislodged, a determination of strength of reaction is made using the criteria described above.
8. The results of the observation are recorded on a worksheet.
9. Steps 2 through 8 are repeated for each of the tubes provided.
10. The results should be checked by the instructor.
11. Readings that are not correct should be repeated.
12. All tubes should be discarded in a puncture-proof biohazard container.

Rouleaux

Agglutination is seen macroscopically as clumping in the tube or on a slide. This agglutination, when seen microscopically, shows random clumps of cells arranged in random patterns. A cellular interaction that macroscopically may mimic agglutination is **rouleaux** (see Figure 2.9). Rouleaux is the cells stacking like coins and does not represent agglutination or an antigen-antibody reaction. Macroscopically in the test tube, this stacking may appear to be agglutination. It may be differentiated microscopically. Rouleaux, when present, is not considered a positive reaction.

COMPLEMENT

Complement is a series of proteins that are activated and involved in immunological reactions. Complement becomes activated in a cascade format. Antibodies to some blood group antigens will cause the activation of complement. This activation may end early in the cascade at the complement component C3. This will

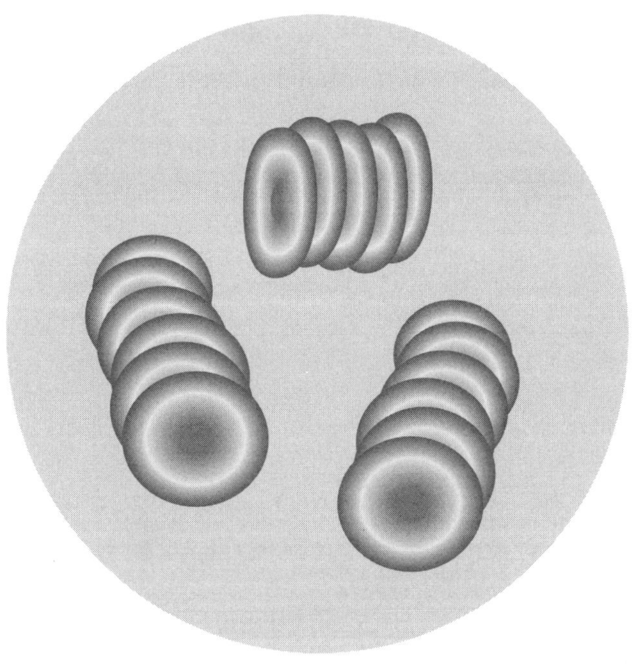

fig. 2.9. Rouleaux.

be detected in the anti-human globulin test. The activation may continue through the entire cascade to C9, resulting in hemolysis of the red cells. The inquisitive student is referred to an immunology text for more information on complement.

ANTI-HUMAN GLOBULIN TEST

The **anti-human globulin (AHG) test** uses an antigen-antibody reaction to detect sensitization or antibody coating the red cells. This AHG test is applied in many test methods in the blood bank. It involves the use of an antibody directed against human globulins to aid in the observation of antigen-antibody reactions.

Some antibodies are capable of making a single attachment to an antigen present on the surface of the cell but are not able to bridge the distance between two red cells to provide a lattice formation and produce agglutination. When the antibodies are unable to bridge cells to produce agglutination, it is necessary to provide assistance in the agglutination process so that positive antigen-antibody reactions may be observed. It is the substance **anti-human globulin (AHG) sera** that provides this bridging effect.

The anti-human globulin test may be divided into two broad categories of tests. These are indirect and direct tests. The **indirect anti-human globulin tests** include all the steps outlined in Table 2.6.

ANTI-HUMAN GLOBULIN REAGENT PREPARATION

Anti-human globulin sera is prepared by injecting an animal (usually a rabbit) with human globulins or antibodies. These human globulins are recognized by

Table 2.6. Method for Using the Indirect Antiglobulin Test

1. Combine sera (or antisera) and cells. Either the sera or the cells comprise the known factor.
2. Centrifuge tubes.
3. Examine, interpret, and record the results.
4. Add enhancement media, if indicated.
5. Incubate 15 to 60 minutes. Be certain not to incubate beyond the 60-minute limit, as the antigen-antibody complexes may begin to dissociate.
6. Centrifuge tubes.
7. Examine, interpret, and record results.
8. Wash tubes three or four times (see Exercise 13).
9. Add AHG sera.
10. Centrifuge tubes.
11. Examine, interpret, and record results.
12. Add Coombs control cells to all negative tubes.
13. Centrifuge tubes.
14. Examine, interpret, and record results.

the animal as foreign. They have the size and biochemical composition to serve as antigens. The rabbit is stimulated to produce antibodies to these human globulins. The substance produced is known as anti-human globulin (AHG) sera. The abbreviation AHG will be used throughout this manual. This reagent is sometimes known as **Coombs' sera**. It is best to avoid the use of that terminology since test methods and other reagents may involve the use of the term "Coombs'" and create confusion.

When preparing AHG sera, the manufacturing process may create different types of sera. These are summarized in Table 2.7. **Polyspecific AHG** contains a mixture of antibodies, whereas the monospecific varieties contain a single type of antibody.

INDIRECT ANTIGLOBULIN TESTING

The indirect method of anti-human globulin testing usually combines a known antigen or antibody with either sera or cells that have an unknown component. After combining the reactants, the test is centrifuged and examined. The tests are incubated at 37°C to facilitate the combination of antigen and antibody. After incubation, the tubes are again centrifuged and examined. Following this step, the tubes are washed three or four times, the saline decanted between each wash, and completely decanted after the final wash. This washing phase dilutes and removes antibodies not bound to the antigens on the red cells. This washing may be performed either manually, using a serological centrifuge, or with an auto-

Table 2.7. Types of AHG Sera

- Polyspecific
  Anti-IgG
  Anti-IgM
  Anti-IgA
  Anti-C_3 (complement)
- Anti-IgG (monospecific)
- Anti-C_3 (monospecific)

mated cell washer. An automated cell washer is pictured in Figure 2.10. Exercise 13 summarizes this washing procedure.

In the final procedural step, the anti-human globulin (AHG) sera designated by the procedure is added in an effort to bridge cells that have become coated with antibodies but are unable to agglutinate. The tubes are centrifuged and examined. See Figure 2.11 for a pictorial summary of the indirect antiglobulin test.

This test is indirect because the cells are coated with antibody **in vitro.** This is compared to the direct antiglobulin test that detects cells coated with antibody **in vivo**. The indirect test is used to determine the presence of either antibodies or antigens. Applications of the indirect AHG test and the direct antiglobulin test will be discussed in Unit 6.

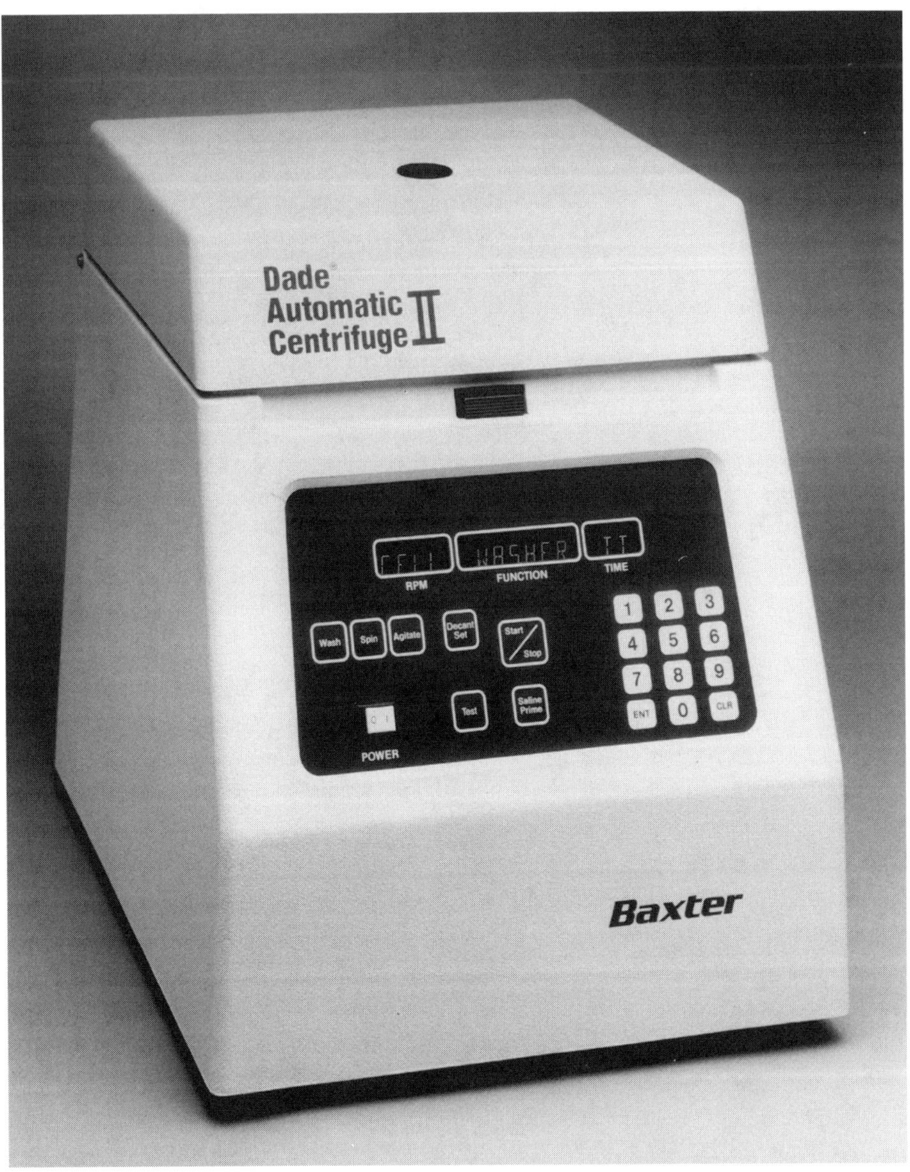

fig. 2.10. Automated cell washer. (Courtesy of American Dade, Division American Hospital Supply Corporation.)

EXERCISE 13 WASHING FOR THE ANTI-HUMAN GLOBULIN PROCEDURE

Each student should practice this washing procedure until determined competent by the instructor.

Equipment:
Gloves
Goggles
10 × 75 or 12 × 75 mm test tubes
Transfer pipets
0.85% saline in a wash bottle
5% suspension of red cells
Laboratory marker
Serological centrifuge
Gauze or laboratory tissues
Beaker with disinfectant
Puncture-proof biohazard container

Procedure:

1. Label two tubes with patient identification.
2. Wearing gloves and goggles, place a drop of 5% cell suspension into each tube.
3. Using the wash bottle, add saline to these tubes to approximately two-thirds full. This saline should be forcefully added to ensure mixing. Be certain not to contaminate the dropper of the wash bottle.
4. Place the two tubes in the centrifuge. Be certain that the centrifuge is balanced.
5. Spin the tubes for 1 minute or the amount of time designated for a wash spin.
6. Remove the tubes when the centrifuge comes to a complete stop.
7. Completely decant the tubes by quickly turning them upside down over the beaker of disinfectant. DO NOT IMMEDIATELY TURN THE TUBES BACK TO AN UPRIGHT POSITION. While still inverted, shake the tubes several times to remove the saline.
8. Return tubes to an upright position. Mix.
9. Repeat steps 3 through 8 two or three additional times. On the third wash, remove the excess saline by blotting the opening of the tubes with either a piece of gauze or some laboratory tissues before returning to an upright position. This provides a "dry button."
10. Dispose of all biohazardous waste in a puncture-proof biohazard container.

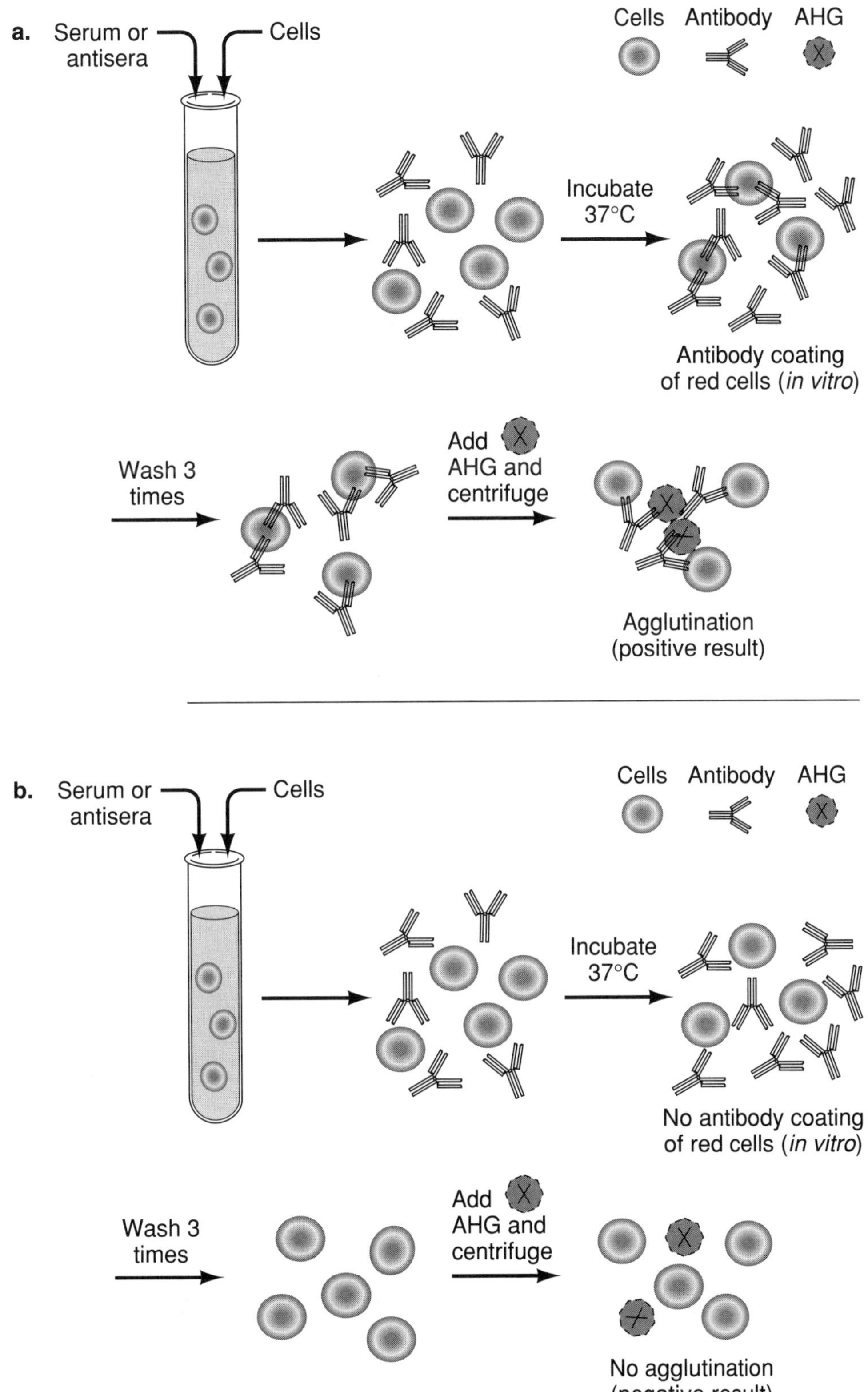

fig. 2.11. Indirect antiglobulin test. a. positive result; b. negative result.

Confirmation of Negative Results

If the tubes are negative, confirmation of these results is necessary. An antibody-coated cell is added as a form of quality control. These cells are called **Coombs' control cells** or **check cells.** Check cells are commercially prepared human group O positive cells coated with anti-D. To prevent confusion with other reagents, this manual will refer to them as check cells.

After adding a drop of coated cells to each negative tube, the tubes are centrifuged and examined. Agglutination should be seen. See Figure 2.12 for a pictorial explanation.

This step confirms that test procedures were performed in a manner that left the unused anti-human globulin sera viable. It also proves that it was not neutralized by human globulins not washed away in the wash phase. Table 2.8 summarizes errors that may cause check cells not to agglutinate.

APPLICATIONS OF THE ANTI-HUMAN GLOBULIN TEST

The anti-human globulin method has many test applications. These applications of the indirect method include the antibody screen test, antibody identification panel, compatibility testing (also known as crossmatching), and antigen typing. These applications will be discussed in later units.

Table 2.8. Errors Causing Check Cells to Present with Negative Results

- Contaminated AHG sera
- Neutralized AHG sera
- Not adding AHG sera
- Dilution of AHG sera
- Not washing serum/cell mixture prior to adding AHG sera
- Inadequate washing of cells
- Contaminated check cells

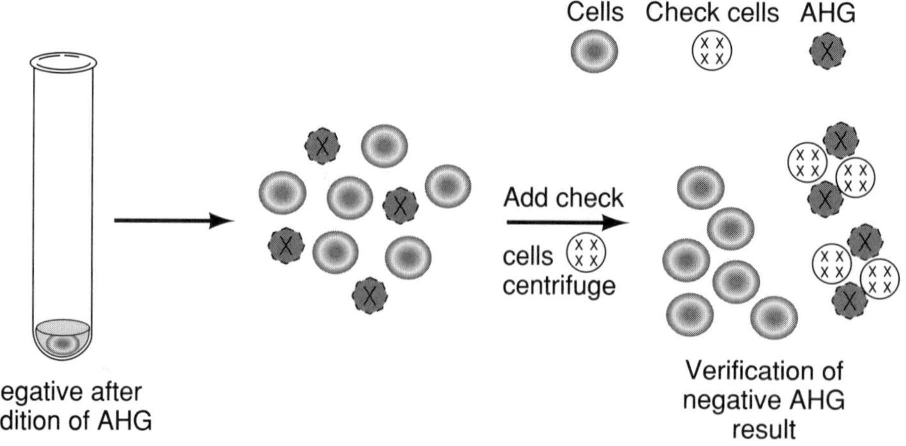

fig. 2.12. Confirmation of negative results with check cells.

GENETICS

The blood group antigens are inherited in the same manner as an individual's other characteristics. The antigen inheritance follows the laws of genetics as defined by Gregor Mendel. Each individual receives one gene from each parent for each of the blood group antigens. The antigens tend to be **codominant.** When two *different* genes are inherited at the same loci on a pair of chromosomes, *both* of these genes will be expressed. For example, when an individual inherits an A gene from one parent and a B gene from the other parent, the expressed blood type will be AB. The applied concepts of genetics will be expanded and discussed in individual sections of the text, as necessary.

SUMMARY

Antigens and antibodies are the principal components of reactions and test procedures in the blood bank. Structure and function of both antigens and antibodies provide the basis for these and other laboratory tests. Antibodies are stimulated by red cell antigens. The red cell antigens that stimulate antibodies are those foreign to the individual. Some antibodies are significant in testing prior to transfusion and during pregnancy. Identification of these antibodies aids the technician in providing blood that is safe for transfusion and diagnosis of hemolytic disease of the newborn and other clinical conditions.

Antigen-antibody reactions are visualized by hemagglutination and hemolysis in the blood bank. The reactions of these antigens and antibodies are evaluated using the same scale in most procedures. Antigen-antibody reactions that cannot be directly visualized may need the addition of anti-human globulin sera to bridge the distance between adjacent red cells. This procedure uses an antibody to human globulins known as anti-human globulin sera. The anti-human globulin method has applications in different test procedures. These procedures will be outlined in later units.

The practical applications of immunology and genetics are many in blood bank testing. Genetics provides the basis for determining antigens present on cells.

The basic concepts presented in this unit will provide the reader with material to apply in future reading and exercises. Understanding and applying this material will be useful throughout the remaining units in the manual.

REVIEW QUESTIONS

1. Which of the following is *not* one of the characteristics of an antigen?
   a. foreign
   b. protein
   c. Y-shaped
   d. complex
2. An IgM molecule is a
   a. monomer
   b. dimer
   c. trimer
   d. pentamer
3. The factors influencing antigen-antibody reactions are varied. In order for the combination of antigen and antibody to be most effective, the reaction temperature is
   a. not important
   b. always room temperature
   c. always 37°C
   d. the optimal temperature
4. When grading an agglutination reaction, the technician notes a cell button breaking away from the bottom of the tube with one gentle shake. It remains intact as one solid clump. This reaction should be graded as
   a. negative
   b. 1+
   c. 2+
   d. 3+
   e. 4+
5. The lag phase of a reaction is that phase where the antibody titer is
   a. undetectable
   b. increasing logarithmically
   c. constant and detectable
   d. declining
6. Secondary antibody stimulation results in a reaction that is termed
   a. anamnestic
   b. a plateau
   c. graphic
   d. primary
7. Zeta potential is the
   a. primary antibody reaction
   b. secondary antibody reaction
   c. net negative cell charge
   d. lattice formation

8. Anticoagulated specimens produce a liquid called
   a. plasma
   b. serum
   c. clotted
   d. agglutinated
9. A natural antibody has been stimulated by a (an)
   a. known antigen
   b. complement component
   c. coagulation factor
   d. unknown antigen
10. Rh immunoglobulin is an example of an antibody that is
    a. actively stimulated
    b. passively stimulated
    c. actively administered
    d. passively administered
11. Anti-human globulin is
    a. directed against red cell antigens
    b. an antibody to human globulins
    c. derived from antibody coated cells
    d. produced in humans
12. Monospecific AHG is
    a. directed against one red cell antigen
    b. reactant with any human globulins
    c. specific for one type of immunoglobulin
    d. always specific for complement
13. The wash phase in the antiglobulin test serves the purpose of
    a. removing the antibody from the red cell surface
    b. diluting the strength of the cell suspension
    c. changing the concentration of the AHG sera
    d. removing the excess serum antibodies

UNIT 3

ABO Blood Group System

LEARNING OBJECTIVES

After studying this unit, it is the responsibility of the student to know the following objectives:

- Define terms listed in the glossary.
- List all antigens and antibodies associated with the ABO blood group system.
- State frequencies of each of the ABO blood groups.
- Discuss the relationship of the H antigen to the ABO blood group system.
- Perform ABO forward and reverse groupings and A_1 subgroupings.

GLOSSARY

amorph gene that does not produce a detectable product.

Bombay phenotype phenotype that possesses no H antigen; designated O_h.

genotype sum total of the genes on the chromosomes.

lectin seed extract that has antibody specificity.

Mendelian as defined by Gregor Mendel; one gene in a pair is inherited from each parent.

neutralization combination of two substances where one has the capability to combine with and render the other inactive in future reactions.

nonsecretor individual who genetically does not produce soluble antigens to be released into the body fluids.

phenotype characteristics detectable with testing.

secretors individuals who have a gene causing soluble forms of antigens to be released into the body fluids.

specificity state of having a certain nature or action.

transferase enzyme that transfers one molecule to another molecule.

INTRODUCTION

The ABO blood group system was discovered in 1900 by Karl Landsteiner. Using the blood of his colleagues, he mixed the serum of some with the cells of others. This led him to discover three of the four ABO groups: A, B, and O. Two years later, some of his pupils discovered the fourth blood group, AB.

ABO grouping is one of the primary tests performed in the blood bank. It is instrumental in pretransfusion testing because it provides the basis for choosing blood for transfusion. Additional test situations that include ABO grouping are prenatal, presurgical, and paternity testing.

This unit will focus on the ABO blood group. Procedures such as forward and reverse grouping will be provided. Many of the principles discussed in this unit will encompass the basic principles in Unit 2.

ABO ANTIGENS

As discussed in the previous unit, the majority of antigens considered in blood bank testing are located on the surface of the red blood cell. The ABO antigens are no exception. When Landsteiner performed his mixing tests, it was these antigens that he was detecting. ABO antigens have been studied at length, and their nature is known in detail.

ABO antigens are also present on the surface of red cells as well as tissue and endothelial cells in the body. In addition, they are found in soluble form in the plasma and other body secretions in a percentage of people known as secretors. Secretor status will be described in more detail later in this unit.

INHERITANCE OF ABO ANTIGENS

ABO antigens are inherited in a simple **Mendelian** fashion from an individual's parents. Each person possesses a pair of genes. One gene of the pair is located on each number 9 chromosome. There are three possible genes that can be inherited. The genes are: A, B, and O. The A and B genes produce a detectable product. The O gene is considered an **amorph,** since it does *not* produce a detectable product. The inherited genes are expressed to form the blood groups that can be determined with testing. Table 3.1 provides a summary of the gene combinations and their expression as blood groups.

It is important to distinguish the terminology associated with the inheritance of blood groups. Table 3.1 describes **genotypes** and **phenotypes** associated with each of the inheritance patterns. Genotype refers to the genes present on the

Table 3.1. Gene Combinations for ABO Blood Group Determination

Blood Group	Gene Combinations
A	AA or AO
B	BB or BO
O	OO
AB	AB

chromosomes, for example AA or AO. It often is not possible to determine the actual ABO genotype for an individual without knowing the blood group of the parents. In comparison, the term phenotype refers to the blood group determined with testing. For example, either genetic pair AA or AO would create the phenotype A. Figure 3.1 demonstrates a grid method for determining parental blood types or offspring types from known or suspected genotypes.

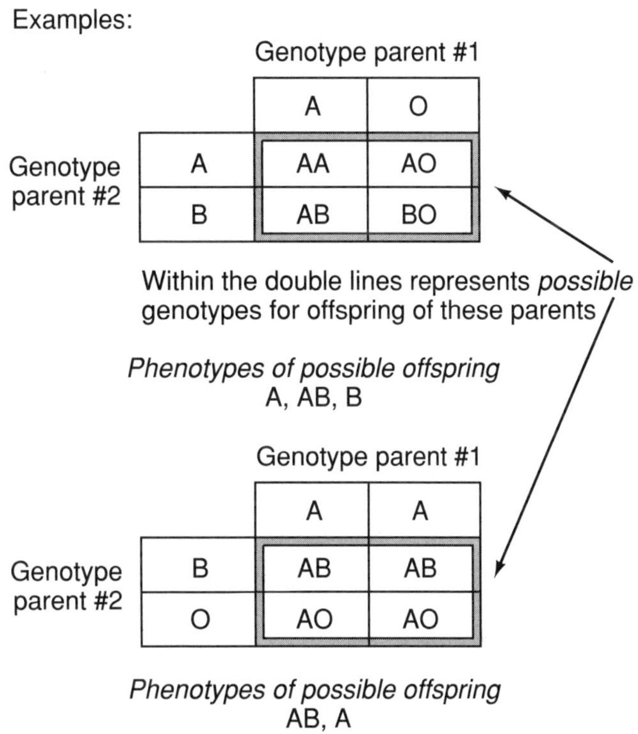

fig. 3.1. Grid method for determining genotypes.

EXERCISE 14 DETERMINATION OF POSSIBLE GENOTYPES FOR OFFSPRING

Using the grid method, determine all possible genotypes for offspring when the parents have the following phenotypes:

1. Father A; Mother O
2. Father AB; Mother B
3. Father B, Mother O
4. Father O, Mother O
5. Father A, Mother B

The A and B genes do not directly produce antigens. Rather they produce an enzyme known as a **transferase**. Each transferase attaches a sugar molecule to the chemical structure of the antigen. It is this sugar molecule that gives the antigen its **specificity**. The O gene codes for no transferase and hence no antigen is produced.

A and B antigens may be found on the surface of red cells or in secretions of those persons who are secretors. The biochemical structure will be the same either on cells or in secretions. When the antigens are on the surface of the red cells, they protrude from the outermost layer of the cell membrane (see Figure 3.2).

To test for these antigens, antisera that is specific for that antigen is used. This antisera contains the specific antibody that will react with the antigen. The A and B antigens are detected either in a test tube or on a slide using the forward grouping test. These test methods will be outlined later in this unit.

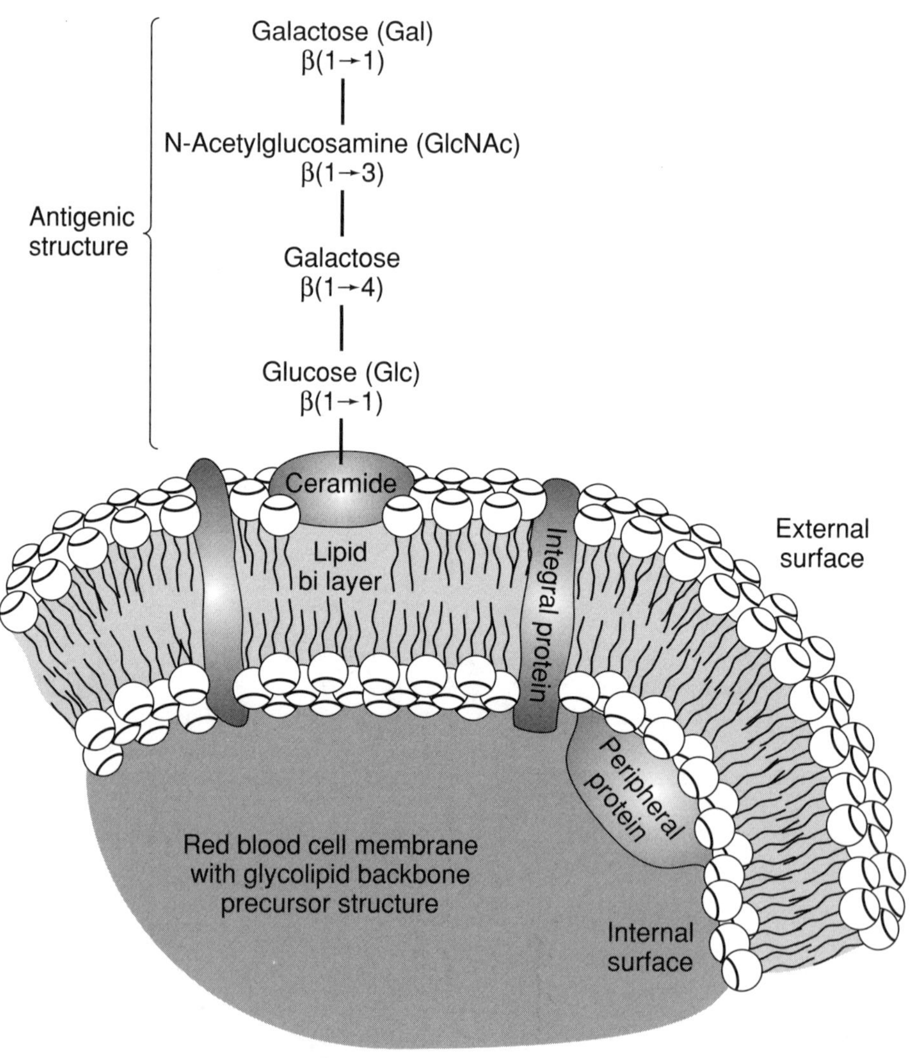

fig. 3.2. Antigen protruding from the surface of the red blood cell.

H ANTIGENS

The H antigen is required to produce either A or B antigens. This antigen is also inherited in a simple Mendelian fashion. Each parent contributes one gene, either H or h. The possible genetic combinations are HH, Hh, or hh. Those individuals who are genetically either HH or Hh will produce the H antigen, and it can be detected on their red cells. The frequency of occurrence of the H antigen in the Caucasian population is greater than 99.99%. The H gene produces a transferase for the addition of a sugar molecule that produces the active antigen.

The H antigen is detected using a specific antisera. This antisera originates from a **lectin** or seed extract known as *Ulex europaeus.* This is not a routine test procedure and will not be discussed further.

The individuals who are hh do not produce the H antigen and have the **Bombay phenotype.** It is represented with the designation O_h. These individuals are very rare and may not be encountered during the course of an entire career working in the blood bank. For additional information on the Bombay phenotype, the more inquisitive student is referred to a textbook on immunohematology.

ABO FORWARD GROUPING

As described previously, the ABO antigens are present on the surface of the red cells whereas the antibodies are found in the serum or plasma. Testing for these antigens and antibodies is performed routinely as a forward and reverse grouping consecutively.

The forward grouping or test for antigens is done by testing the patient's cells containing unknown antigens with known antisera. This antisera contains an antibody specific for the antigen being tested. For example, anti-A will combine with the A antigen. These antisera are manufactured from human sera and should be treated as a biohazard. The test is performed using a suspension of 2% to 5% washed patient cells. The procedure for preparing a 5% cell suspension washed cell suspension is as follows:

EXERCISE 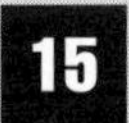

PREPARATION OF SUSPENSION OF PATIENT'S WASHED RED BLOOD CELLS

Each student should be given an anticoagulated specimen to prepare the cell suspensions. The student should note that in the blood bank the use of a clotted sample is standard. An anticoagulated sample is being used in this exercise for ease of handling. A clotted sample may be used if the instructor desires.

Equipment:
Gloves
Goggles
10 × 75 or 12 × 75 mm test tubes
Transfer pipets

EXERCISE 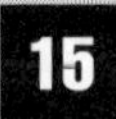

PREPARATION OF SUSPENSION OF PATIENT'S WASHED RED BLOOD CELLS *(continued)*

Serological centrifuge
Test tube rack
Isotonic saline (0.85%–0.90%) in a wash bottle
Small beaker with isotonic saline
Large beaker with disinfectant
Marking pen
Laboratory tissues
0.1 ml serological pipet or 100 µl micropipet
5.0 ml serological pipet
Safety bulb
Parafilm
Puncture-proof biohazard container

Part I: Preparing an Exact 5% Washed Red Cell Suspension

1. Label three test tubes as follows:
   Plasma/patient identification
   Washed cells/patient identification
   5% cell suspension/patient identification

NOTE: *Labeling is a critical step in any laboratory procedure and should be done carefully.*

2. Centrifuge the blood sample, if necessary.
3. Wearing gloves and goggles, use a transfer pipet and carefully remove the "Plasma" to the labeled tube.

NOTE: *Be careful not to contaminate with red cells.*

4. When most of the plasma has been removed, remove some red cells from the bottom of the patient sample tube and place them in the tube labeled "Washed Cells".

NOTE: *This tube should be no more than half full of cells.*

5. Forcefully add saline from the wash bottle to the "Washed Cells" tube until the liquid level is about ½ inch from the top.

NOTE: *Be careful not to contaminate the tip of the wash bottle dispenser with blood. See Figure 3.3.*

6. Cover the top of the tube with parafilm and invert to mix.
7. Centrifuge with a balance tube for 1 minute at 3400 rpms. See Figure 3.4.

EXERCISE 15 PREPARATION OF SUSPENSION OF PATIENT'S WASHED RED BLOOD CELLS *(continued)*

NOTES: *Never open the lid of the centrifuge before the spinning action has come to a complete stop. The spin time may vary on individual centrifuges. The student should check the calibration information for the centrifuge in use.*

8. Discard parafilm into the biohazardous waste.
9. Using a transfer pipet, carefully remove the supernatant and discard it into the large beaker with disinfectant. Be certain not to splash any of the supernatant or disinfectant on the counter.
10. Repeat steps 5 through 9 two more times. This makes a total of three washes.

NOTE: *During these washing steps, procedure step #11 may be done in the interest of time efficiency.*

11. Using the 5.0 ml pipet and a safety bulb, pipet 1.9 ml of saline from the small beaker into the tube labeled "5% cell suspension."
12. Using the 0.1 ml pipet (or micropipet) and a safety bulb, add 0.1 ml of patient's cells to the saline in the "5% cell suspension" tube.
13. Cover with parafilm and mix. This is an *exact* 5% cells suspension.
14. Discard all biohazardous waste in a puncture-proof biohazardous waste container.

Part II: Preparing an Approximate 5% Washed Cell Suspension

1. Label two test tubes as follows:
   Washed cells/patient identification
   5% cell suspension/patient identification
2. Wearing gloves and goggles, perform steps 4 through 10 from the procedure for preparing an exact 5% washed red cell suspension.
3. Using the tube labeled "5% cell suspension," fill the tube half full with isotonic saline from the wash bottle.
4. Using a transfer pipet, add cells from the "washed cell tube" until the color and concentration of cells in the tube is approximately the same as the exact cell suspension prepared in the previous procedure.
5. Dispose of all biohazardous waste into a puncture-proof biohazard container.

NOTE: As the cells are added, use the transfer pipet to mix the solution by rinsing the pipet with the saline/cell mixture in the tube. This transfer pipet may then be used to transfer the 5% cell mixture into the tubes to be tested.

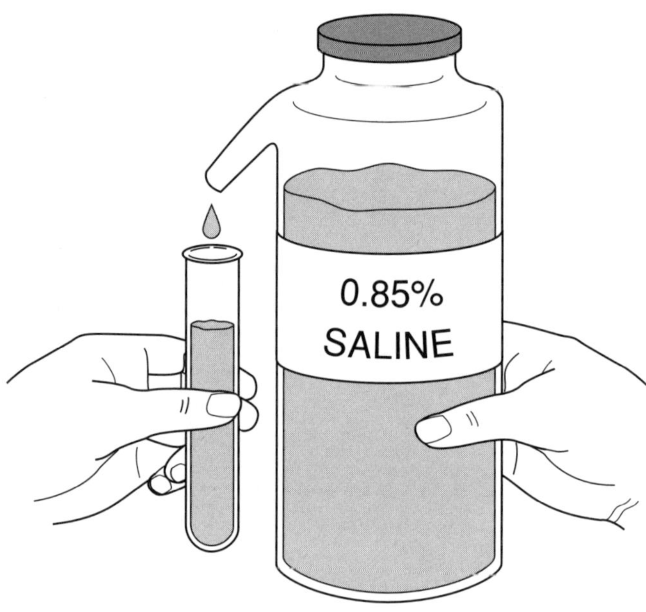

fig. 3.3. Saline should be added to test tubes without contaminating the wash bottle. This is done by adding the saline without placing the tip of the wash bottle into the tube.

When performing the forward ABO grouping, an approximate 2% to 5% cell suspension is used. The preceding exercise includes an activity for preparing an exact 5% cell suspension. This was done so that each student may use this exact suspension as a standard for comparison when preparing the approximate 5% cell suspension.

ANTISERAS

Three antiseras are available for ABO forward grouping. These antiseras are summarized in Table 3.2. The forward grouping may be performed using all three or, in the case of patients, only the anti-A and anti-B are used. For the purposes of reinforcement of theory, the procedure included in this manual will use all three antiseras.

These antisera will be reacted in a 1:1 ratio with the patient's 2% to 5% cell suspensions when performing the tube typing. Test results for each blood group are summarized in Table 3.3. When evaluating these test results, the antigens on the cells are reacting with the specific antibodies in the antisera. It is this reaction that produces the visible agglutination. Examining this table, it is clear that a group A individual has the A antigen that will react with both anti-A and anti-A,B, whereas group O reacts with no antisera because these cells have neither A nor B antigens.

Table 3.2. Antiseras for ABO Forward Grouping

Antisera	Color	Source
Anti-A	Blue	Group B donor
Anti-B	Yellow	Group A donor
Anti-A,B	Clear	Group O donor

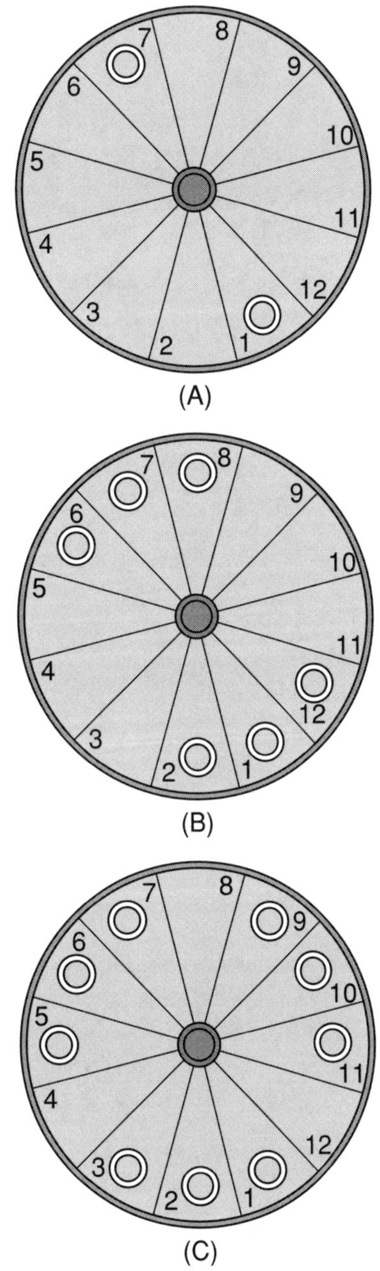

fig. 3.4. A centrifuge is balanced by placing two tubes in directly opposite tube slots.

Table 3.3. Reaction Patterns for ABO Groups

Blood group	Anti-A	Anti-B	Anti A,B
A	Positive	Negative	Positive
B	Negative	Positive	Positive
AB	Positive	Positive	Positive
O	Negative	Negative	Negative

EXERCISE 16 EXAMINATION OF ABO ANTISERA

Students should divide into small groups. Each group will be given the following equipment:

Equipment:
Gloves
Goggles
Anti-A antiserum
Anti-B antiserum
Anti-A,B antiserum
Package inserts from each antiserum

Each group of students should:

1. Wearing gloves and goggles, examine each bottle of antisera to determine the color of the three antisera. This information should be recorded.
2. Each vial of antiserum should be examined to be certain that it is clear and no debris is floating in the vial. The condition of each vial should be recorded.

NOTE: *Cloudy antisera or free-floating debris implies that the antisera is contaminated and should be discarded into a puncture-proof biohazardous waste container.*

3. Check the expiration date. Record this expiration date and the lot number of each vial.
4. Read the package insert for each antiserum. Determine the type of antibody present in each and the source of each antiserum. Record this information.
5. Locate any warnings regarding the biohazardous nature of these antisera. Read and follow these warnings.
6. Have an instructor check your work.

The use of anti-A,B antiserum is significant to note. This antisera is obtained from an individual who is group O. It is not a mixture of anti-A and anti-B, but rather a separate antibody that will react with both the A and B antigens. It is used in the forward grouping for two purposes:

1. It confirms the results of the anti-A and anti-B (see Table 3.3).
2. It will show a positive reaction, with weak subgroups of A and B that do not react with the anti-A and anti-B. (The more inquisitive student is referred to a textbook on immunohematology for more information on reactions of subgroups with anti-A,B).

The procedure for ABO forward grouping is presented in Exercises 17 and 18. ABO forward grouping is most often done in test tubes (Tube Typing), but may be done on glass slides (Slide Typing).

EXERCISE 17 ABO FORWARD GROUPING: TUBE TYPING METHOD

For this procedure, each student should use an approximate 2% to 5% cell suspension. The suspension prepared in Exercise 15 may be used.

Equipment:
Gloves
Goggles
Serological centrifuge
10 × 75 or 12 × 75 mm test tubes
Transfer pipets
Isotonic saline in a wash bottle
Antiseras (anti-A, anti-B, anti-A,B)
Test tube rack
Marking pen
Beaker with disinfectant
Agglutination viewer lamp
Puncture-proof biohazardous waste container

Procedure:

1. Wearing gloves and goggles, prepare an approximate 5% cell suspension using the procedure in Exercise 15.
2. Label three test tubes with the patient's name and identification number.
3. Each of these tubes should then be labeled as follows:
   First tube: "Anti-A"
   Second tube: "Anti-B"
   Third tube: "Anti-A,B"

NOTE: Labeling should be done with care since clerical errors are the most frequent errors in the blood bank.

4. Check clarity and expiration date on antisera; record information.
5. To each of these tubes, add 1 drop of the corresponding antisera.

NOTE: Use a free falling drop.
Do not touch the dropper to the side of the tube.
Always add antisera before cells.

6. Using a transfer pipet, add 1 drop of the well-mixed 5% cell suspension to each of these three tubes.

EXERCISE 17 ABO FORWARD GROUPING: TUBE TYPING METHOD *(continued)*

NOTE: Use a free falling drop.
Do not touch the pipet to the side of the tube.

7. Gently mix all tubes.
8. Centrifuge all three test tubes for 15 seconds at 3400 rpm.

NOTE: Time may vary with each centrifuge. Check the calibration information for each individual centrifuge. Never open the lid of the centrifuge before the spinning motion stops.

8. Gently resuspend each tube and look for hemolysis and agglutination in the manner described in Unit 2.
9. Grade each reaction and record the results.
10. Have the instructor check your work.
11. Dispose of all biohazardous waste in a puncture-proof container.

EXERCISE 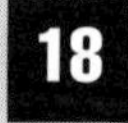 18 ABO FORWARD GROUPING: SLIDE TYPING METHOD

Each student will need an anticoagulated blood sample to perform this exercise. For performing slide grouping, a whole blood sample is used. This provides approximately a 50% cell suspension. This exercise may also be performed on blood from a capillary puncture if desired.

Equipment:
Gloves
Goggles
3 × 5″ plain glass slides
Transfer pipets
Antisera (Anti-A, Anti-B, Anti-A,B)
Wooden applicator sticks
Grease marking pencil
Marking pen
Stopwatch
Puncture-proof biohazard container

Procedure:

1. Mark three slides by drawing an oval in the center of the slide (see Figure 3.5).

EXERCISE **18** ABO FORWARD GROUPING: SLIDE TYPING METHOD *(continued)*

NOTE: A typing slide may be used. If this is the case, the oval markings will already be on the slide.

2. Each slide should also be marked "Anti-A," "Anti-B," or "Anti-A,B."
3. Wearing gloves and goggles, on each slide place 1 drop of the corresponding antisera inside of the circle.
4. Mix the blood sample until all cells have been suspended in the plasma.

NOTE: If a capillary specimen is to be used directly from the puncture site, the puncture should be performed at this time. Be certain to use all safety procedures during the capillary collection.

5. In each circle, place a drop of whole blood next to the drop of antisera.
6. Mix antisera and cells within the circle using an applicator stick.
7. Start a stopwatch
8. Rock the slide gently for 2 minutes. Look for agglutination using a strong light.
9. Record as "+" for agglutination and "0" for negative.
10. Repeat using the next slide.
11. Interpret the results when all three slides have been read.
12. Call the instructor to check the results.
13. Dispose of all biohazardous waste in a puncture-proof waste container.

SUBGROUPS OF A AND B ANTIGENS

The A and B antigens may be further divided into subgroups. A subgroup is a variation in the antigen that makes it different from other subgroups, but still chemically the same antigen. Many subgroups exist for the A blood group. The two principal ones are A_1 and A_2. The B subgroups are rare and will not be discussed in this manual.

A_1 AND A_2 ANTIGENS

The A_1 and A_2 subgroups are the most frequently encountered. These subgroups are inherited in the manner described previously. Approximately 80% of group A individuals are group A_1, with A_2 comprising most of the remaining percentage. A very small percentage of group A persons are a subgroup other than A_1 or A_2. There are qualitative and quantitative differences in the subgroups.

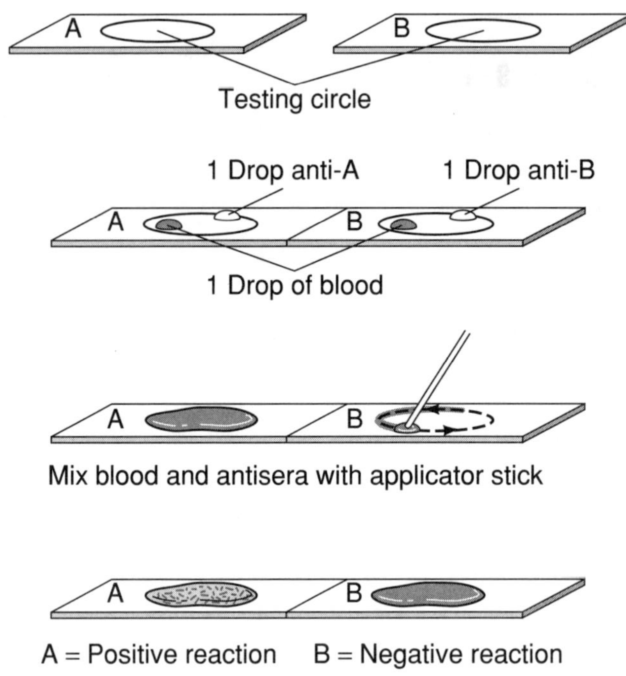

fig. 3.5. Slide typing for ABO forward grouping.

The most significant difference between A_1 and A_2 subgroups is that an A_2 or A_2B individual may develop an antibody to the A_1 antigen. In this case, the individual will show a forward group of A or AB while the reverse group will show agglutination with the A_1 cells.

The differentiation of A_1 and A_2 cells can be made with an antisera specific for the A_1 antigen. This antisera is known as anti-A_1 lectin or A_1 lectin. The most common form is prepared from the extract of a seed known as *Dolichos biflorus*. This antisera will give a positive reaction with A_1 cells and will show no reaction with A_2 cells or those cells from other subgroups of A. When performing this test, proper controls must be run to determine the accuracy of the antisera. Known A_1 and A_2 cells are tested as positive and negative controls, consecutively. The procedure for testing group A cells for A_1 antigen is outlined in Exercise 19.

ABO ANTIBODIES

The ABO blood group provides the only situation in which *each* individual produces antibodies corresponding to antigens not present on the surface of the red cells. ABO antibodies are natural antibodies formed with no apparent antigenic stimulus. The antigenic stimulus is environmental, and exposure occurs following birth.

Newborns have no ABO antibodies of their own. When newborns are tested, only a forward group is performed. They may have antibodies that have passively crossed the placental barrier. If the serum of a newborn or the umbilical cord serum *is* tested, the results will most likely indicate the blood group of the mother. The child will begin to produce antibody and have a detectable titer at

EXERCISE 19 SUBGROUPING OF GROUP A CELLS

Each student will be given one or more group A samples to test.

Equipment:
Gloves
Goggles
Serological centrifuge
Anti-A_1 antisera
10 × 75 or 12 × 75 mm tubes
Transfer pipets
Beaker with disinfectant
Test tube rack
Marker
Isotonic saline in a wash bottle
Puncture-proof biohazard container

Procedure:

1. Wearing gloves and goggles, the student should prepare an approximate 5% cell suspension for each of the samples. See Exercise 15 for the cell suspension preparation procedure.
2. Label three test tubes:
   Patient/identification
   Positive control
   Negative control
3. Into each of these three tubes place 1 drop of the anti-A_1 antisera.
4. Using a transfer pipet, place 1 drop of the patient's 5% cell suspension into the patient's tube.
5. Into the positive control, place 1 drop of A_1 reverse grouping cells.
6. Into the negative control, place 1 drop of known A_2 cells.
7. Centrifuge all tubes for 15 seconds at 3400 rpm.

NOTE: Centrifuges will vary in their centrifugation time. Check the calibration readings for the centrifuge being used.

8. Using an agglutination viewer, gently resuspend each tube, observing for hemolysis and agglutination.
9. Record results on a worksheet.
10. Have the instructor check the results.
11. Discard all tubes and biohazardous waste into a puncture-proof biohazard container.

about 6 months of age. Other instances of low level ABO antibody titers are summarized in Table 3.4.

ABO antibodies detectable in the plasma or serum are antibodies that *do not* correspond to the antigens on the surface of the cells. This follows Landsteiner's law stating that an individual does not normally develop antibodies to antigens found on the surface of their red cells. For a summary of the antibodies found in each blood group, refer to Table 3.5.

These antibodies are characteristically IgM antibodies reacting at room temperature after an immediate spin. There may also be a mix of IgG antibodies in the serum. It is this IgG fraction of the antibodies that would have the ability to cross the placenta and cause hemolytic disease of the newborn. Hemolytic disease of the newborn will be discussed in a later unit.

The test for ABO reverse grouping uses patient serum containing unknown antibodies. The serum is combined with cells having known antigen content in a 2:1 ratio. The result is evaluated by examining the tubes for hemolysis and agglutination and grading the reactions. The standard reverse grouping reagents are commercially prepared saline suspended A_1 and B cells. These cells are of human origin and should be considered a biohazard. The interpretation of the four blood groups in the reverse group test are summarized in Table 3.6.

Remember that when making blood group interpretations the antibodies present in the serum are those corresponding to antigens not on the surface of the cells. For example, Group A has the A antigen and will have the corresponding B antibody. When the serum is reacted with the reagent red blood cells, the B antibody will react with the antigens on the B cells, but not those on the A cells. Therefore, a positive reaction will be seen in the B tube, but not in the A tube (see Table 3.6).

Table 3.4. Conditions with Decreased Levels of ABO Antibodies

- Newborns and young infants
- Elderly individuals
- Immunodeficient individuals
- Immunosuppressed patients

Table 3.5. Antigens and Antibodies in ABO Blood Groups

Blood Group	Antigens	Antibodies
A	A	Anti-B
B	B	Anti-A
O	Neither A nor B	Anti-A and anti-B
AB	A and B	Neither anti-A nor anti-B

Table 3.6. Interpretation of Reverse Grouping Test Results

Blood Group	A_1 Cells	B Cells
A	Negative	Positive
B	Positive	Negative
O	Positive	Positive
AB	Negative	Negative

Anti-H is a rare antibody encountered in only a very small percentage of the population, since most individuals have the H antigen. This antibody is found most often in individuals with the Bombay phenotype.

EXERCISE 20 ABO REVERSE GROUPING

Each student will perform this test on the plasma from the specimen evaluated in Exercise 17. Each student should have one blood sample that has been separated into cells and plasma. The tube typing method for forward grouping and this exercise are routinely performed concurrently. After students have become proficient in each of the two activities, they should be encouraged to perform them simultaneously.

Equipment:
Gloves
Goggles
Serological centrifuge
10 × 75 or 12 × 75 mm test tubes
Transfer pipets
Isotonic saline in a wash bottle
Marking pen
Beaker with disinfectant
A_1 and B cells
Agglutination viewer
Puncture-proof biohazardous waste container.

1. Label two test tubes with patient's name and identification number.
2. Label one of these tubes A and the second B.

NOTE: Labeling is a crucial step in the blood typing procedure. Fatal errors are made when clerical errors occur.

3. Wearing gloves and goggles, add 2 drops of serum to each tube.
4. To the appropriate tube, add 1 drop of well-mixed reagent red cells.

NOTE: Before using these reagent red cells, be certain that they are mixed and that all of the cells are resuspended from the bottom of the vial.

5. Gently mix the two tubes.
6. Centrifuge for 15 seconds at 3400 rpm.

NOTE: The time for centrifuging may vary with the individual centrifuge. Be certain to check the calibration on the centrifuge that is being used.

7. Remove each tube and examine for hemolysis.

EXERCISE 20 ABO REVERSE GROUPING *(continued)*

8. Using an agglutination viewer, gently resuspend each cell button and examine for agglutination.
9. Grade each reaction and record on a worksheet along with the Forward Grouping performed in Exercise 17.
10. Have the instructor check all results.
11. Discard all tubes and biohazardous waste into a puncture-proof biohazardous waste container.

SECRETOR

As previously mentioned, ABO antigens are found on red cells and tissue cells throughout the body as well in the secretions of some individuals. Approximately 80% of individuals will have soluble ABO antigens in their body fluids. These individuals are known as **secretors.**

Secretor status is determined by the inheritance of a gene known as the secretor gene. This gene is inherited in a Mendelian fashion, with one gene of the pair coming from each parent. The possibilities are "Se" or "se." An individual who inherits either one or two "Se" genes will have the capability to produce soluble antigens secreted into the body fluids. The inheritance of two recessive "se" genes will result in a **nonsecretor** status, where no soluble antigens will be secreted into the body fluids.

The secretor status may be determined by using saliva. The test employs the combination of soluble antigens with the antibodies in standard typing sera. When cells specific for the antigen are added, there will be *no reaction* if a soluble antigen was present. An agglutination reaction will occur if no soluble antigen was present in the saliva. This type of test is known as a **neutralization** test. A textbook on immunohematology will discuss secretor status in more detail.

FREQUENCIES OF ABO BLOOD GROUPS

The four blood groups exist in given frequencies within a population. Various references state slightly different frequencies for the individual blood groups. An approximation of the frequencies is summarized in Table 3.7.

Table 3.7. Frequencies of ABO Blood Groups

Blood Group	Frequency
O	45%
A	41%
B	10%
AB	4%

SUMMARY

The ABO blood group system is the backbone of blood bank testing. The ABO antigens were first discovered by Landsteiner and still play a prominent role in pretransfusion, prenatal, and presurgical testing. The H antigen system is vital to the understanding of the ABO biochemistry. Individuals may also secrete a soluble form of the A, B, and H antigens into the body fluids. Detection of secretor status may be tested using saliva.

Forward and reverse grouping is performed routinely in even the smallest blood bank. The accuracy of this test is important to a successful transfusion experience for the patient.

Group A antigens may be divided into subgroups, with A_1 being the most frequent. The A_1 antigen may be detected using a specific antisera. This test is significant since an individual with another subgroup may develop an antibody to the A_1 antigen. This antibody will be detectable in testing.

The basic principles of antigens and antibodies have been applied to the ABO system in this unit. The technician must have an understanding of the ABO system and the methods of testing. Test methods for detection of antigens and antibodies in this system are similar to those used to test other blood groups. Some of these principles will be applied in other units throughout this manual.

CASE STUDY 

An ABO group was performed on the cord blood of a full-term healthy infant. The mother was O Rh negative. The following results were obtained:

Anti-A	*Anti-B*	*Anti-A,B*	*A cells*	*B cells*
4+	0	4+	4+	4+

QUESTIONS

1. What is the ABO group of this baby? Explain your response.
2. Are any discrepancies noted in these results?
3. How does the test procedure vary from what you would expect for a newborn? Why?
4. Does knowing the blood group of the mother help to explain the results?

CASE STUDY 2

A presurgical patient has been tested to determine the blood group in case a transfusion is necessary during surgery. The results of the ABO grouping are as follows:

Anti-A	*Anti-B*	*Anti-A,B*	*A cells*	*B cells*
4+	0	4+	2+	4+

QUESTIONS

1. What is the ABO group of this patient? Explain your response.
2. Are any discrepancies noted in these results? Explain.
3. What could have caused this situation to occur?
4. In your opinion, have errors occurred in testing? Explain.

REVIEW QUESTIONS

1. A forward group is performed, with the following results:

Anti-A	*Anti-B*	*Anti-A,B*
4+	0	4+

   The expected results for the reverse grouping would be
   a. A cells—positive; B cells—positive
   b. A cells—positive; B cells—negative
   c. A cells—negative; B cells—positive
   d. A cells—negative; B cells—negative
2. The Bombay phenotype is comprised of a genetic combination of
   a. O_h
   b. HH
   c. Hh
   d. hh
3. The notation of AO represents a
   a. Bombay phenotype
   b. genotype
   c. phenotype
   d. transferase
4. An individual presents with the following typing results:

Anti-A	*Anti-B*	*Anti-A,B*	*A_1 cells*	*B cells*
4+	0	4+	1+	4+

   This individual is
   a. group AB
   b. group A_2 with anti-A_1
   c. group A_1 with anti-A
   d. unable to determine

5. Anti-H is found in the sera of individuals of group
   a. A
   b. B
   c. O
   d. O_h
6. Parents of group A and AB *cannot* produce offspring of group
   a. A
   b. B
   c. AB
   d. O
7. If a group A individual reacts 3+ with A_1 lectin, this person is a (an)
   a. A_1
   b. A_2
   c. AB
   d. Bombay
8. An individual presents with the following ABO grouping results:

Anti-A	*Anti-B*	*Anti-A,B*	*A_1 cells*	*B cells*
0	4+	4+	4+	0

   This individual is group
   a. A
   b. B
   c. AB
   d. O
9. Of the following choices, the individual with a potential for having a reduced amount of ABO antibody is a
   a. blood donor
   b. recently immunized adult
   c. newborn
   d. postsurgical patient
10. Anti-A antisera comes from an individual who is group
   a. A
   b. B
   c. AB
   d. O

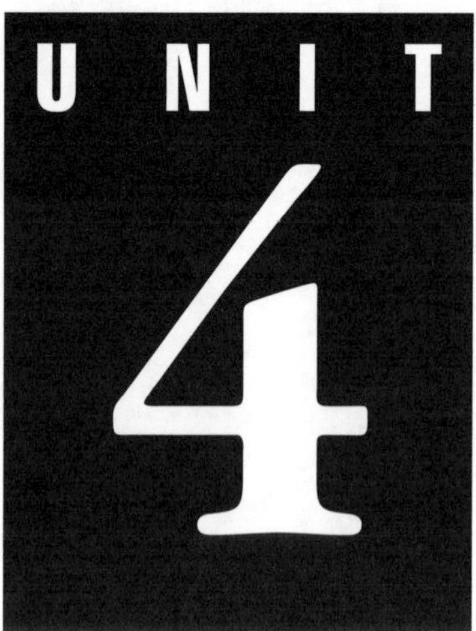

Rh Blood Group System

LEARNING OBJECTIVES

After studying this unit, it is the responsibility of the student to know the following objectives:

- Define terms listed in the glossary.
- List the Rh antigens and describe their inheritance.
- Outline the characteristics of antibodies to the Rh antigens.
- Discuss the weak D antigen.
- Describe and perform the procedure for testing for the Rh_o(D) and weak D antigen.
- Determine the most probable Rh genotype.

GLOSSARY

allele paired gene for any given gene on a chromosome.

locus location of a gene on a chromosome.

monoclonal antisera antisera where the antibodies are derived from a single clone of cells.

recipients individuals who receive a transfusion of blood or its components.

Rh null phenotype with a lack of Rh antigens on the surface of the red cells.

steric related to the spatial arrangement of the molecules.

sublocus location within the gene locus.

INTRODUCTION

The Rh blood group system is the second most recognized blood group. The notation accompanies the ABO group in blood type designation. Donors are identified by the ABO and Rh antigen status. Blood components for transfusion are also labeled in that manner. Rh_o(D), the major Rh antigen, plays a vital role in hemolytic disease of the newborn and will be discussed in that role later in this manual.

The Rh blood group system includes additional red blood cell antigens. The inheritance of these antigens will be outlined in this unit.

RH ANTIGENS

As with the ABO system, the Rh antigens are located on the surface of the red blood cells. In contrast to the ABO system, Rh antigens are found exclusively on the red cells and are not found on tissue cells or in soluble form in the body fluids.

The biochemical nature of the Rh antigens is lipoprotein. These antigens are an integral part of the red cell membrane, compared to the ABO antigens, which protrude from the outermost layer of the red cell membrane. This antigenic characteristic plays a part in testing methods for antigens.

RH_0(D) ANTIGEN

The Rh_o(D) antigen is the primary antigen in the system. When present on red cells, the individual is designated as Rh positive. This antigen will be called the "D" antigen throughout the remainder of this manual. The notation Rh_o(D) will be explained in a section later in this unit.

The D antigen is inherited as a Mendelian characteristic from an individual's parents. This inheritance is slightly different than that of the ABO antigens. The D gene is located on the number 1 chromosome. An individual may inherit one D gene from each parent. The inheritance of either one or two D genes will designate that person as "Rh positive." The incidence of Rh positive persons is 85% in the white population and 92% in the African-American population.

If one parent does not contribute a D gene, there is no other gene that is contributed. Originally, it was believed that a "d" gene existed and could serve as the matching gene, or **allele** for the D gene. This d gene was never discovered. Consequently, when no D gene is inherited from either parent, the individual is designated as "Rh negative." Rh-negative individuals comprise about 15% of the white population and 8% of the African-American population (see Table 4.1).

Table 4.1. Frequency of Occurrence of the Rh Antigens

Antigen	% in White Population	% in African-American Population
D	85	92
C	70	33
c	80	97
E	30	21
e	98	99

Testing for the Rh_0(D) Antigen

To test for the D antigen, an antisera containing antibodies specific for the D antigen is used. This antisera is designated "anti-D." The antibody contained in the antisera will attach to the D antigen on the patient's or donor's cells and cause agglutination if the cells have this antigen. The tube test is similar to that for the ABO antigens. A 2% to 5% suspension of washed red cells is used for testing in a 1:1 ratio with the antisera. The antisera originates from a human source and should be considered a potential biohazard.

Compared to the ABO antisera, the antisera used to test for the D antigen has different constituents. Whereas the ABO antisera are diluted and suspended in saline, anti-D is available in different forms. These forms of anti-D are summarized in Table 4.2. Quality control and procedures for use will differ for each of these typing sera. When using any antisera, the package inserts for the specific reagents should be consulted.

Since the antigens are an integral part of the cell membrane and are less numerous than the ABO antigens, it is more difficult for the antibody molecules to attach and form the lattice needed for agglutination. The use of high protein media reduces the zeta potential and allows the cells to agglutinate on immediate spin. Chemical modification of the immunoglobulin molecule allows the hinge region of the molecule to span greater distance to attach to antigen-binding sites. This enhances the ability of the antibody to attach to antigens and agglutinate. The use of **monoclonal antisera** has expanded. The origination of the antibody is from one antibody-producing clone and is very specific.

Historically, high-protein antisera was used in parallel with a control. Chemically modified antisera is readily available, and the use of a parallel control is no longer necessary. Since the use of chemically modified antisera provides a clear positive or negative reaction without the interpretation of a parallel control, explanation of its use is minimal. In the interest of clinical or student laboratories using a high-protein media, a discussion of the use of this media with a parallel control will be included.

When using the high-protein media for Rh typing, a control is performed with each patient sample. This control assures that the agglutination obtained in the patient test represents a true positive reaction. The control known as "Rh control" is composed of contents identical to the anti-D sera, but with no antibody. When used in parallel with the patient test, this control should always be negative. If the control tube is positive, the test is considered invalid. When a positive control is obtained, the technician must determine the reason for the positive result. Reasons for invalid tests are numerous. The inquisitive student is referred to an immunohematology textbook for further explanations of invalid controls.

When performing an Rh control with the test, it is important to use Rh control reagent from the same manufacturer as the anti-D sera that is being used. This assures that the constituents of the Rh control solution are identical to that

Table 4.2. Categories of Anti-D Typing Sera

High Protein Anti-D—antisera in which an IgG form of anti-D is diluted and suspended in a high-protein media

Chemically Modified Anti-D—IgG anti-D that has been modified by chemical treatment and suspended in a media with a protein concentration similar to human serum

Monoclonal Anti-D—mixture of monoclonal IgG and IgM anti-D having a protein concentation similar to that of human serum

IgM Anti-D—IgM anti-D suspended in saline media

EXERCISE **21**

EXAMINATION OF Rh ANTISERA AND Rh CONTROL

Equipment:
Gloves
Goggles
Anti-D antisera
Rh control
Package inserts for anti-D and Rh control

1. Wearing gloves and goggles, examine the anti-D sera and the Rh control.
2. Check the expiration date and lot number and record.
3. Examine the antisera and control to be certain that they are visually clear and contain no floating debris. Record your observations.
4. Discard any solutions that are cloudy or have floating debris into a puncture-proof biohazard container.
5. Read the package inserts for both reagents. Determine how to use them and any special precautions to be made when handling these reagents.
6. Have the instructor check your work.

EXERCISE 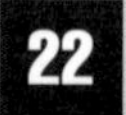

Rh TYPING OF RED BLOOD CELLS BY THE TUBE METHOD

For the following exercise each student should be given either a clotted or an anticoagulated blood sample. Note that, in the blood bank, clotted specimens are most often used for routine testing. This procedure uses a chemically modified antisera. If a high protein antisera is used, a parallel control should be used and tested in the same manner as the test.

Equipment:
Gloves
Goggles
10 × 75 or 12 × 75 mm test tubes
Transfer pipets
Test tube rack
Marking pen
Chemically modified anti-D antisera
0.85% saline in a wash bottle
Serological centrifuge

EXERCISE 22 Rh TYPING OF RED BLOOD CELLS BY THE TUBE METHOD *(continued)*

Agglutination viewer
Puncture-proof biohazard container
Beaker with disinfectant

Procedure:

1. Wearing gloves and goggles, prepare a 2% to 5% suspension of the patient's red blood cells as outlined in Exercise 15.
2. Label a test tube with patient identification and "anti-D."

NOTE: The labeling of tubes is a crucial step in the procedure and should be done with care.

3. To the tube, add 1 drop of antisera.

NOTE: For step 3, be careful not to contaminate the dropper by being certain that it does not touch the inside of the tube. Also, do not lay the dropper on the counter or other surface. Return the dropper to the bottle immediately.

4. Using a transfer pipet, add 1 drop of the patient's cell suspension to the tube.
5. Centrifuge for 15 to 30 seconds, as designated by the manufacturer.

NOTE: Spin time will vary with centrifuge. Check the calibration for the centrifuge being used. Never open the lid of the centrifuge until all the parts have stopped moving.

6. Resuspend the cells by gentle agitation and examine under a good light source for agglutination.
7. Record and interpret results immediately.
8. Dispose of all biohazardous waste into a puncture-proof biohazardous waste container.

in the anti-D, with the exception of the antibody. This typing may be performed either by a tube or slide method.

Weak D

The D antigen may appear in some individuals in a weakened form. Historically, this weakened form was referred to as the D^u variant. Throughout this manual, this antigen will be called the "weak D." This weakened form of the D antigen may be caused by one of three situations.

The first situation is one in which a piece of the D antigen is missing. The D antigen is a mosaic by structure and composed of several pieces. If one or more of these pieces are missing, the antigen is present in its modified form.

The second scenario is one in which the D gene is on a chromosome opposite a C gene. This placement presents a **steric** hindrance and will not permit the D antigen to be produced in the same quantity as when the C antigen is not blocking its production (see Figure 4.1). The C gene is said to be in the "trans" position to the D gene. In contrast, the "cis" position would be the two genes, for example D and C, located on the same chromosome.

The final case involves the inheritance of a gene that codes for less D antigen. This genetic inheritance occurs less frequently than the other two methods of inheritance and is most often encountered in African-Americans.

Testing for the weak D. When the weak D is present, initial Rh typing will appear as Rh negative. The test is taken through further steps to enable the antigen, if present, and antibody additional time and optimal conditions to become attached and to demonstrate a positive reaction. This requires completion of the anti-human globulin procedure. The theory for this procedure was discussed in Unit 2.

Additional testing for the weak D includes incubating the test at 37°C for 15 to 60 minutes to facilitate the formation of the antigen-antibody complex. When the weakened antigen is present, the attachment of antibody occurs during the incubation. The antibody molecules are not wide enough to form complexes with the antigens on other cells. Therefore, agglutination does not occur at this point in the testing.

After incubation, the tubes are filled with saline, centrifuged, and decanted three to four times in an effort to "wash" away all of the excess antisera and proteins. The final step is to add anti-human globulin sera to bridge the antibody molecules attaching to the antigens on the red cells (see Figure 4.2).

Interpretation of the test for the weak D antigen is made when all testing is complete, but prior to the addition of the check cells. A positive test indicates that there is D antigen present on the surface of the cells. This antigen is present in a weakened form, but these individuals still possess the antigen and are considered Rh positive in some instances.

Individuals who have a weak D are considered Rh positive for the purposes of donating blood for transfusion. For this reason, the test for the weakened D antigen is still performed routinely as a part of donor testing. On the other hand, individuals who are to receive a blood transfusion or **recipients** are considered

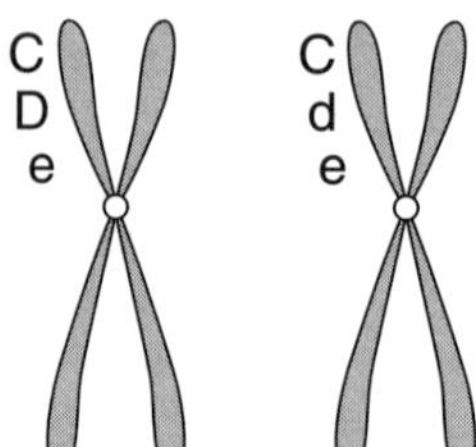

fig. 4.1. Weak D, where the "C" gene is in the "trans" position to the "D" gene on the opposite chromosome.

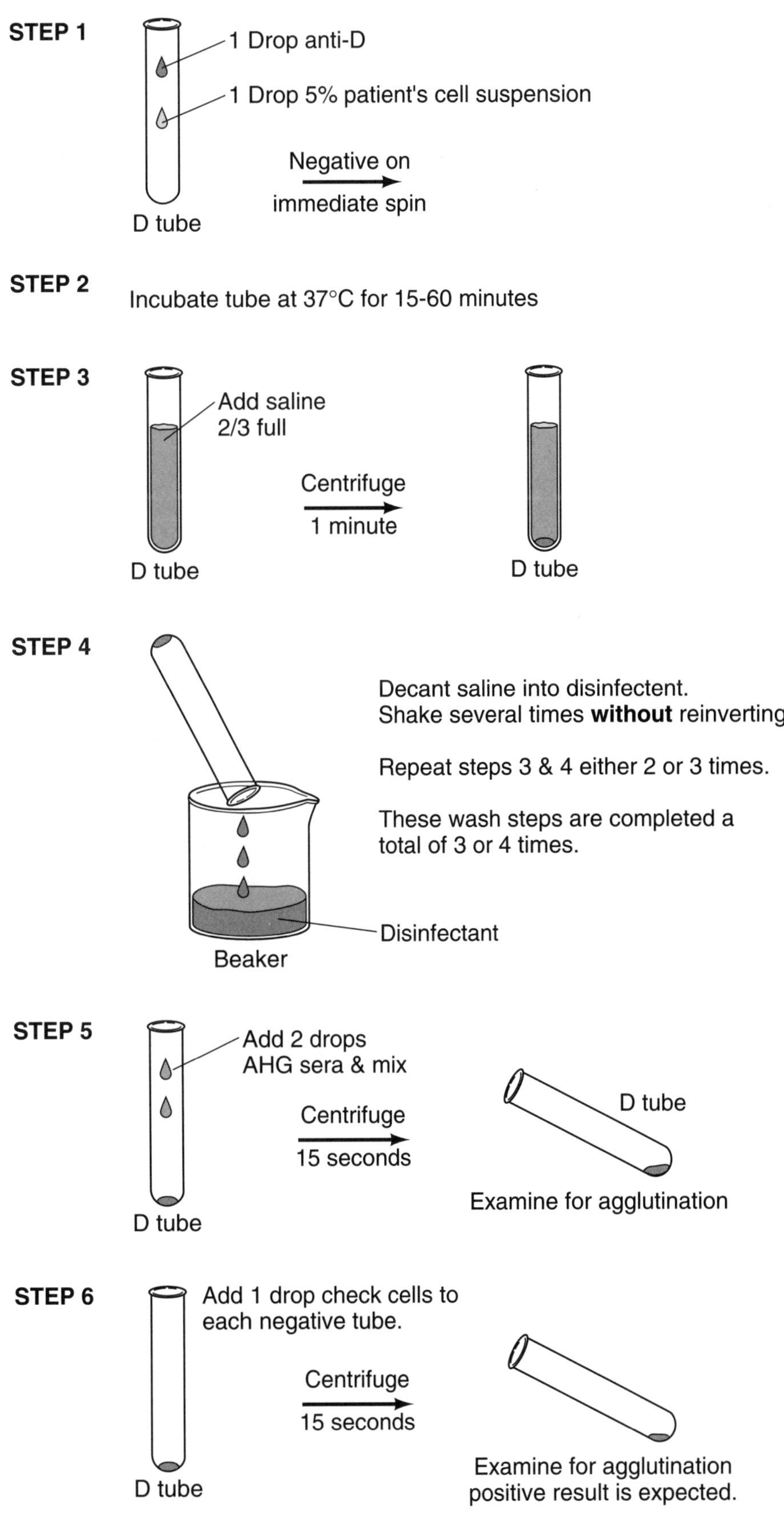
STEP 1
1 Drop anti-D
1 Drop 5% patient's cell suspension
Negative on
immediate spin
D tube
STEP 2
Incubate tube at 37°C for 15-60 minutes
STEP 3
Add saline
2/3 full
Centrifuge
1 minute
D tube
D tube
STEP 4
Decant saline into disinfectent.
Shake several times without reinverting.
Repeat steps 3 & 4 either 2 or 3 times.
These wash steps are completed a
total of 3 or 4 times.
Disinfectant
Beaker
STEP 5
Add 2 drops
AHG sera & mix
Centrifuge
15 seconds
D tube
Examine for agglutination
D tube
STEP 6
Add 1 drop check cells to
each negative tube.
Centrifuge
15 seconds
D tube
Examine for agglutination
positive result is expected.

fig. 4.2. Testing for the weak D using the anti-human globulin procedure.

Rh negative if the test for the weakened D antigen is positive. These individuals should receive Rh-negative blood. If the weakened D is caused by a mosaic pattern and the individual is transfused with Rh-positive blood, it is theorized that the individual develops an antibody to the portion of the D antigen that they are missing. Consequently, many institutions have stopped performing the test for the weakened form of the D antigen on most potential recipients. The exception to this is the expectant or postpartum mother. The policies of the institution should be checked by the technician if uncertainty exists.

EXERCISE 23 TEST FOR WEAK D ANTIGEN

Each student should be provided with an Rh-negative sample to perform this test. The sample used for analysis in Exercise 22 is acceptable if it is Rh negative. The procedure outlined below is that for using chemically modified antisera. If a high-protein media is used, a parallel control should be used and treated in an identical manner to the test.

Equipment:
Gloves
Goggles
Serological centrifuge
37°C heat block
Timer
0.85% saline in a wash bottle
Beaker with disinfectant
Agglutination viewer
Anti-human globulin sera
Check cells
Puncture-proof biohazard container

Procedure:

1. Wearing gloves and goggles, place the anti-D tube containing a presumptive Rh-negative sample into the 37°C heat block.
2. Set a timer for 15 minutes.

NOTE: This incubation may extend for up to 60 minutes. If performing additional tests, the timing may be adjusted to suit the workload.

3. When time has elapsed, use the wash bottle of saline to fill the tubes two-thirds full with saline.

NOTE: Be careful not to contaminate the dropper of the wash bottle when dispensing the saline. The dropper should be held in a manner so that it does not extend into the neck of the test tubes.

4. Centrifuge for 1 minute. Remember to check the calibration on the centrifuge and adjust this spin time if the centrifuge requires a different amount of time for washing.

EXERCISE 23 TEST FOR WEAK D ANTIGEN *(continued)*

5. When centrifugation is complete, hold the tube by the bottom and turn upside down over the beaker of disinfectant. While still in the upside down position, shake to remove as much saline as possible. DO NOT TURN UPRIGHT UNTIL YOU HAVE COMPLETED THE DISPENSING OF THE SALINE. If you accidentally turn upright without completely dispensing, DO NOT REINVERT. Continue with the following steps.
6. Gently mix the cells in the small amount of saline remaining.
7. Steps 3 to 6 are repeated either two or three more times for a total of three or four washes. On the final wash, shake the tube hard to dispense as much saline as possible. The lips of the tube may be blotted with a laboratory tissue or paper towel before turning upright. Check with the instructor before doing this. Remember that it creates a biohazard and the tissues or towels should be appropriately discarded.
8. To the tube, add 2 drops of anti-human globulin reagent. Mix.
9. Centrifuge for 15 seconds (or the appropriate amount of time as determined with calibration).
10. Read using an agglutination viewer.
11. Record results.
12. Interpret results as follows:
    D tube negative: Rh negative
    D tube positive: Weak D positive
13. To each negative tube, add one drop of well-mixed check cells. (These should yield a positive result. This implies that the test has been properly performed. Negative results with these cells indicate an improperly performed test and the test should be repeated.)
14. Spin for 15 seconds.
15. Read using an agglutination viewer.
16. Record results.
17. Discard all biohazardous waste into a puncture-proof biohazard container.

CcEe ANTIGENS

Additional antigens that fall under the Rh system are numerous. The only ones to be considered here are the two pairs of alleles: Cc and Ee. The inheritance for these is by Mendelian rules. The genes are inherited by the offspring receiving one gene of each type from each parent. This means that each parent contributes either E or e *and* either C or c, so that the final combination includes two genes from each of the two categories. Some examples of genotypes include CCEE, CcEE, and ccee. Any combinations are possible. Frequency of occurrence for these antigens is summarized in Table 4.1. There are additional Rh antigens, but these are less often discussed and will not be considered further in this unit. The more inquisitive student is referred to an immunohematology textbook.

FISHER-RACE AND WEINER NOMENCLATURES

While the inheritance of these antigens is by Mendelian rules, there have been two major theories of inheritance proposed. A resolution of the correct theory has never been made. The two theories are Fisher-Race and Weiner. Each of these will be presented and explained. The notations are different for the two theories, and it is useful for the student to be able to make the conversions from one system to another.

Fisher-Race Theory of Inheritance

The Fisher-Race theory states that each of the three possible genes that can be inherited from an individual's parents, D, Cc, Ee, originate from a different **locus**. This means that each prospective antigen is produced by a *separate* gene. These three genes are located in very close proximity to each other. In fact, they are so close that it is impossible for any crossing-over to occur and alter the strict Mendelian inheritance of these antigens (see Figure 4.3).

Hence, the genes are inherited as a group. For example, a parent with the genotype DCe/DcE will contribute either the group DCe or DcE to each offspring. The individual genes are not inherited singly, and so the combination Dce could not possibly be inherited from this parent. For example, an offspring from this parent could be DCe/dce, with DCe coming from this parent and dce being contributed by the second parent.

The frequencies of the various combinations of these genes in the populations are summarized in Table 4.3. The frequencies will, again, vary in different populations.

The Fisher-Race terminology has been used throughout this unit. The antigens are referred to by the letters D, C, c, E, and e. Because this terminology is simple to remember and understand, it has been chosen to be the primary system of notations used throughout this manual. That does not mean that it is the true system of inheritance, but rather that it simplifies the understanding and communications for the learner.

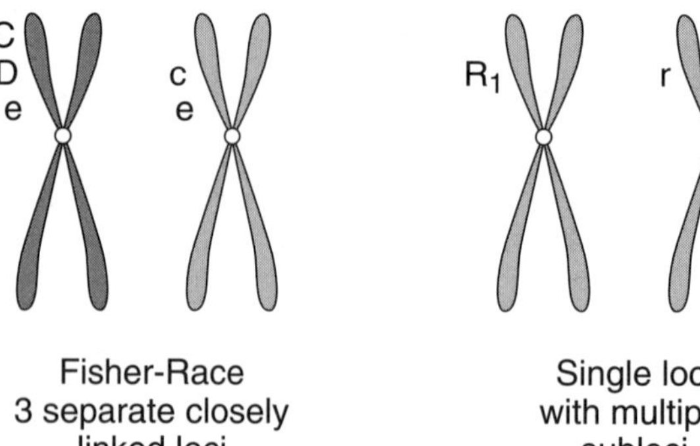

fig. 4.3. Comparison of chromosome placement of genes in the Fisher-Race and Weiner theories of Rh inheritance.

Table 4.3. Frequencies of Fisher-Race Gene Combinations

Fisher-Race Gene Combinations	Weiner Shorthand Notation	Percentage in Whites	Percentage in African-Americans
CDe	R^1	0.42	0.17
cDE	R^2	0.14	0.11
cDe	R^o	0.04	0.44
CDE	R^z	Rare	Rare
cde	r	0.37	0.26
Cde	r'	0.02	0.02
cdE	r"	<0.01	Rare
CdE	r^y	Rare	Rare

Weiner Theory of Inheritance

The theory of inheritance proposed by Weiner and his colleagues differs from the Fisher-Race theory. It states that the Rh antigens are inherited from a *single* locus and that each of the antigens represents a **sublocus** within that single locus. Therefore, the two or three antigens are inherited as a single unit rather than as two or three individual units closely linked, as was proposed by Fisher-Race.

Each gene codes for either two or three factors. These factors correspond to the antigens defined by Fisher-Race. (See Table 4.4 for a summary of the Fisher-Race and Weiner terminology.)

Conversion of Fisher-Race and Weiner Terminologies

It is important to understand the relationship between the Fisher-Race and Weiner terminologies and to be able to make conversions between the two systems both mentally and on paper. At the beginning of this unit, the D antigen was referred to as the Rh_o(D) antigen. This is a combination of Fisher-Race and Weiner terminologies. Throughout the unit, this antigen was called the D antigen for simplicity. For a summary of these conversions see Table 4.5.

Most Probable Genotypes

In the laboratory the technician will perform Rh phenotyping by testing the patient's red cells for antigens with antisera specific for each antigen. Included are tests for the D, C, c, E, and e antigens. For each test, a positive and negative control for each antisera must be included. For example, when testing for the C antigen, a positive control would involve the use of anti-C antisera with red cells that are known to have the C antigen. A negative control would contain the antisera with the cells that are known to be negative for the C antigen. Once these tests for antigens have been completed, the results reflect the phenotype of the patient. The antigens present may be found in different genotype combinations.

Table 4.4. Summary of Fisher-Race and Weiner Terminology

Fisher-Race Antigens	Weiner Factors
D	Rh_o
C	rh'
E	rh"
c	hr'
e	hr"

Table 4.5. Conversions between Fisher-Race and Weiner Nomenclatures

Fisher-Race		Weiner	
Gene Combinations	**Antigens**	**Gene**	**Factors**
DCe	D,C,e	R^1	Rh_o, rh', hr"
DcE	D,c,E	R^2	Rh_o, hr', rh"
Dce	D,c,e	R^o	Rh_o, hr', hr"
DCE	D,C,E	R^z	Rh_o, rh', hr"
dce	c,e	r	hr', hr"
dCe	C,e	r'	rh', hr"
dcE	c,E	r"	hr', rh"
dCE	C,E	r^y	rh', rh"

Frequently, it is impossible to determine which genotype is present without testing the parents and other family members. For this reason, the determination of most probable genotype is usually made by using a table such as Table 4.6. The most probable genotype is the one having the highest percentage of incidence for the antigens present.

Rh NULL

Very rarely an individual will present with a total lack of Rh antigens on the surface of the red cells. These individuals are known as **Rh null**. This occurrence is extremely rare and may not be encountered in an entire career in the laboratory.

Rh ANTIBODIES

Compared to the ABO system, individuals who lack any of the Rh antigens rarely develop antibodies to those antigens without active stimulation. The active stimulation occurs by pregnancy or transfusion.

The characteristics of the Rh antibodies are summarized in Table 4.7. Presence of these antibodies is considered atypical. Testing for these antibodies in the serum is by the antibody screen test. This test will be summarized in Unit 6.

Table 4.6. Antigen Typing Results and Determination of Most Probable Genotypes

Typing Results					Possibilities in Order of Frequency
D	*C*	*E*	*c*	*e*	
+	+	0	+	+	Dce/dce, DCe/Dce, dCe/Dce
+	+	0	0	+	DCe/DCe, DCe/dCe
+	+	+	+	+	DcE/DCe, DCe/dcE, DCE/dce, DCE/Dce, dCE/Dce
+	0	+	+	0	DcE/DcE, DcE/dcE
+	0	0	+	+	Dce/dce, Dce/Dce
0	0	0	+	+	dce/dce
0	+	0	+	+	dCe/dce
0	0	+	+	+	dcE/dce
0	+	+	+	+	dCe/dcE, dCE/dce
0	+	0	0	+	dCe/dCe
0	0	+	+	0	dcE/dcE
+	+	+	0	+	DCE/DCe, DCE/dCe
+	+	+	+	0	DCE/DcE, DCE/dcE
+	+	+	0	0	DCE/DCE, DCE/dCE
0	+	+	0	+	dCE/dCe
0	+	+	+	0	dCE/dcE
0	+	+	0	0	dCE/dCE

EXERCISE 24

DETERMINATION OF MOST PROBABLE Rh GENOTYPES

For each of the following sets of test results, determine the most probable genotype using the statistics in Table 4.6.

Results of Antigen Typing

	D	*C*	*c*	*E*	*e*
1.	+	+	+	+	+
2.	+	0	+	+	+
3.	0	+	+	0	+
4.	0	0	+	0	+

Table 4.7. Characteristics of Rh Antibodies

Immunoglobulin class	IgG
Optimal temperature of reactivity	37°C
Optimal media of reactivity	Albumin/anti-human globulin
Capable of crossing the placenta	Yes
Capable of causing HDN	Yes
Capable of causing hemolytic transfusion reaction (HTR)	Yes

SUMMARY

The Rh system contains antigens that are important in blood bank testing. These Rh antigens are found on the surface of the red cells and are directly inherited from an individual's parents. The D antigen is important for pretransfusion testing as well as predicting and diagnosing clinical conditions such as hemolytic disease of the newborn.

Rh antigens other than the D antigen include C, c, E, and e. These antigens are inherited individually, with one of each pair coming from each parent. Each individual has two genes of each type, so that possible combinations include CC, Cc, or cc and EE, Ee, or ee. Tests to detect these Rh antigens are not performed in routine testing. These antigens are significant. Their corresponding antibodies may be encountered and create problems with transfusion and newborns. Testing for all Rh antigens is performed in a similar manner to the testing for ABO antigens.

Testing for the weak D antigen is done using the anti-human globulin test. Presence of the weakened D is significant in choosing blood for transfusion and labeling donor units. It is theorized that antibodies to the missing portion of the antigen may develop in some instances.

Antibodies to the Rh antigens may be stimulated by transfusion or pregnancy. Rarely are they naturally occurring. They are IgG immunoglobulins and have the ability to cross the placenta. They are implicated in causing hemolytic disease of the newborn and hemolytic transfusion reactions. Detection and identification of serum antibodies within this system are significant and will be addressed with other antigen-antibody systems in Unit 6.

CASE STUDY 3

A female patient is seen in the prenatal clinic and has the standard series of tests normally performed during pregnancy. The blood bank is requested to perform an ABO and Rh and forward the results to the clinic. The technician performing the test achieved the following results:

Anti-A	*Anti-B*	*Anti-D*	*Rh Control*	*A cells*	*B cells*
0	0	2+	2+	4+	3+

QUESTIONS

1. What is the interpretation of the Rh typing results? Explain.
2. What types of circumstances may have caused these results?
3. What is the next step that the technician should take in testing this patient?
4. Using your current knowledge, if transfusion would be necessary, what ABO and Rh type of blood would you choose?

CASE STUDY 4

During testing, a donor tests negative in both the D and Control tubes on immediate spin. The technician continues by testing both tubes with the anti-human globulin procedure. After the addition of the anti-human globulin sera, the following results were obtained:

Anti-D	*Rh Control*
2+	0

QUESTIONS

1. How would you interpret these results? Explain.
2. As a donor, would this person be Rh positive or Rh negative? Why?
3. If this person would receive blood by transfusion, should Rh positive or Rh negative blood be administered? Why?
4. What, if any, further testing needs to be performed on this donor?

REVIEW QUESTIONS

1. The approximate percentage of persons in the white population who are Rh negative is
   a. 15
   b. 25
   c. 50
   d. 85
2. The antigen missing in the Rh negative individual is
   a. C
   b. c
   c. D
   d. d
3. The Weiner notation R_1R_2 translates to Fisher-Race as
   a. DCe/DcE
   b. DCe/DCE
   c. DCE/DcE
   d. DCe/Dce
4. When performing an Rh typing, the results obtained for an Rh-positive individual are
   a. anti-D–positive; Rh control–positive
   b. anti-D–positive; Rh control–negative
   c. anti-D–negative; Rh control–positive
   d. anti-D–negative; Rh control–negative

5. The following test results are obtained:

Anti-D	*Anti-C*	*Anti-c*	*Anti-E*	*Anti-e*
0	+	+	0	+

   The most probable genotype is
   a. R_1r
   b. R_or
   c. r'r
   d. rr
6. Formation of Rh antibodies is stimulated by
   a. environmental substances
   b. proteins
   c. ABO antibodies
   d. transfusions
7. The weak D antigen is
   a. identical to the D antigen
   b. missing part of the D antigen
   c. an Rh-negative antigen
   d. not at all related to the D antigen
8. The weak D may be created when the D antigen is
   a. absent on both chromosomes
   b. inherited from only one parent
   c. in the trans position to the C gene
   d. received in an Rh-positive transfusion
9. Fisher-Race describes the inheritance of the Rh antigens as resulting from
   a. one locus with three subloci
   b. a single complete unit
   c. three separate closely linked loci
   d. linkage to the ABO genes
10. In the test for the weak D, the AHG sera serves the purpose of
   a. enhancing antibody attachment to the D antigen
   b. bridging antibody molecules attached to red blood cells
   c. reducing zeta potential
   d. diluting antisera

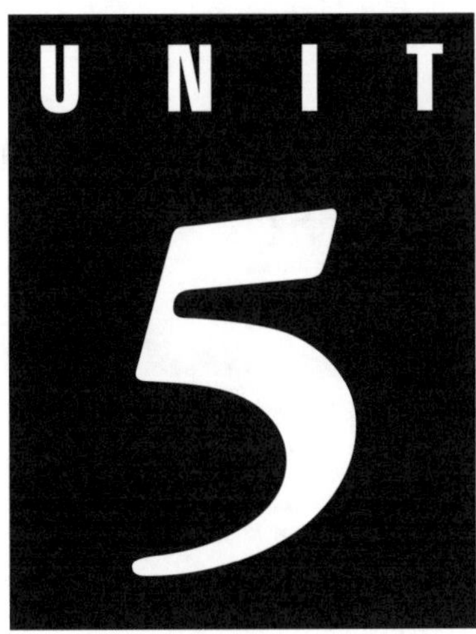

Other Blood Group Systems

LEARNING OBJECTIVES

After studying this unit, it is the responsibility of the student to know the following objectives:

- **Define terms listed in the glossary.**
- **List blood group systems and antigens contained in each system.**
- **Discuss the characteristics of the antibodies that correspond to each of the antigens.**
- **Relate the methods of antibody stimulation for each of the antigen-antibody systems discussed.**
- **Perform at least one antigen typing at room temperature and one using an anti-human globulin procedure.**

GLOSSARY

dosage characteristic of an antibody to react stronger with cells that have a homozygous presentation of the antigen.

titer strength of an antibody defined by serially diluting the antibody and reacting it with its antigen at each dilution; weakest dilution showing a positive reaction is the titer.

universal antigen antigen found on the red cells of a large percentage of the population, approaching 100%.

INTRODUCTION

In previous units, two major antigen systems have been discussed. There are additional antigen systems which each contain multiple antigens that may be found on the surface of the red cells. Each individual does not possess all possible antigens. The antigens present on the cells of each person are determined by inheritance.

Antibodies to these antigens, while not normally present, may be formed by an individual who is exposed to the antigen and does not have that antigen on the surface of their red cells. The exposure to antigens occurs either during pregnancy or blood transfusion. Some antibodies may be formed naturally without direct stimulation.

Antigens of the major systems, as well as antibodies corresponding to each of those systems, will be discussed briefly in this unit. The characteristics of the various antibodies will be outlined and should be considered important for the remaining units in this manual. The antigen-antibody systems will be broadly categorized by optimal temperature of reactivity and individual systems discussed in each of these categories. Testing for these antibodies will be discussed in the test procedures outlined in Unit 6, "Testing for Unexpected Antibodies."

SYSTEMS WITH COLD-REACTING ANTIBODIES

Antigen systems to be discussed in this section are summarized in Table 5.1. The antibodies formed tend to react at room temperature (25°C) or colder. The technician must be aware that temperatures of reactivity are not always the same for a given antibody. Some antibodies that are usually IgM cold-reactive antibodies may also develop as IgG warm-reactive antibodies. This classification has been made for the sake of organization, but should not be considered as strict rules for the performance of the antibodies. Identification of antibodies will be discussed in Unit 6.

Antibodies that react best at temperatures less than body temperature (37°C) are not considered clinically significant since any reactions seen in the test tube will most likely not be seen at the warmer temperatures of the body. For that reason, whereas the antibodies may be encountered in testing and identified when performing the appropriate testing, they are not likely to cause a transfusion-related accident.

Table 5.1. Antigen Systems with Cold-Reacting Antibodies

System	Major Antigens
Lewis	Le^a, Le^b
P	P_1
I	I, i
MNSs	M, N, S, s

LEWIS BLOOD GROUP SYSTEM

The Lewis system is a system containing two major antigens, Le^a, Le^b (pronounced "Lewis a" and "Lewis b"). The frequencies of these antigens are summarized in Table 5.2.

These antigens differ from most antigens since they are not initially found on the surface of the red cell. They are formed in the secretions and absorbed onto the surface of the cell later. The mechanism for determining the final cell type is complex. The inquisitive student is referred to a textbook of immunohematology for a more detailed explanation.

Lewis Blood Group Antibodies

Lewis antibodies are most often encountered in individuals with no Le^a or Le^b antigens. These individuals are described with the notation Le(a-b-) (pronounced "Lewis a negative, b negative"). Characteristics of the antibodies are summarized in Table 5.3. These antibodies are often IgM cold-reacting, although some IgG anti-human globulin-reacting varieties are seen. They may be formed naturally without direct stimulation. Lewis antibodies are characterized by the fact that they may be present at certain times, such as during pregnancy, and then disappear. They are not threatening to a transfusion recipient's welfare unless they react at anti-human globulin phase or cause hemolysis in the test process.

MNSs BLOOD GROUP ANTIGENS

Like many other systems, the MNSs system is composed of numerous antigens. The most frequently discussed are M, N, S, s, and U. Frequencies for these antigens are summarized in Table 5.2. M and N act as a pair of alleles, with either M or N inherited from each parent. This provides the possibility of having a final genotype of *MM, MN,* or *NN.* S and s act as a second pair of alleles, with one being inherited from each parent. Final possibilities for genetic combinations are *SS, Ss,* and *ss.*

Therefore, the final genetic component of each individual will consist of two genes from the MN group and two from the Ss group. For example, a possible genotype would be *MMSs.*

The U antigen is a **universal antigen** found in the majority of individuals. This antigen is found whenever either S and/or s antigens are present.

MNSs Blood Group System Antibodies

Antibodies to the MN antigens are most often cold-reacting antibodies of the IgM classification. These antibodies may be naturally occurring or stimulated by direct exposure. The antibodies will display the **dosage** effect. In this case, the weakened antibody will react more strongly with cells that possess a stronger antigen. For example, a cell that is genetically MM may react with a 2+ reaction whereas a cell that is MN will only react 1+. These test results may be confusing at first, but careful examination will aid in the interpretation.

In contrast, antibodies to the Ss antigens are most often reactive at 37°C and at the anti-human globulin phase of testing. This temperature of reactivity does remove these antibodies from the cold-reacting category, but they are considered here since they are related to the M and N antigens. All of these antibodies are summarized in Tables 5.3 and 5.4.

Table 5.2. Antigen Frequencies in Adults

Antigen	Frequency (%)	
Le^a	White 22	African-American 23
Le^b	White 72	African-American 55
P_1	White 79	African-American 94
M	White 78	African-American 70
N	White 72	African-American 74
S	White 55	African-American 31
s	White 89	African-American 97
K	White 9	African-American 2
k	White 99	African-American >99
Jk^a	White 77	African-American 91
Jk^b	White 72	African-American 41
Fy^a	White 66	African-American 10
Fy^b	White 83	African-American 23

Table 5.3. Characteristics of Cold-Reacting Antibodies

Antibody	Ig Class	Optimal Temp*	Optimal Media*	Causes HDN†	Causes HTR‡
Anti-Le^a	IgM	25°C	Saline	No	No
Anti-Le^b	IgM	25°C	Saline	No	No
Anti-M	IgM	25°C	Saline	No	No
Anti-N	IgM	25°C	Saline	No	No
Anti-S	IgG	37°C	AHG§	Yes	Yes
Anti-P_1	IgM	25°C	Saline	No	No
Anti-I	IgM	25°C	Saline	No	No
Anti-i	IgM	25°C	Saline	No	No

*Optimal means where most examples react.
†Hemolytic disease of the newborn.
‡Hemolytic transfusion reaction.
§Anti-human globulin.

Table 5.4. Characteristics of Warm (AHG)-Reacting Antibodies

Antibody	Ig Class	Optimal Temp*	Optimal Media*	Causes HDN†	Causes HTR‡
Anti-K	IgG	37°C	AHG§	Yes	Yes
Anti-k	IgG	37°C	AHG	Yes	Yes
Anti-Jk^a	IgG	37°C	AHG	Yes	Yes
Anti-Jk^b	IgG	37°C	AHG	Yes	Yes
Anti-Fy^a	IgG	37°C	AHG	Yes	Yes
Anti-Fy^b	IgG	37°C	AHG	Yes	Yes
Anti-s	IgG	37°C	AHG	Yes	Yes

*Optimal means where most examples react.
†Hemolytic disease of the newborn.
‡Hemolytic transfusion reaction.
§Anti-human globulin.

P_1 ANTIGEN AND ANTI-P_1

The P blood group system is composed of four antigens with the P_1 antigen being the definitive antigen. The inheritance for this antigen is slightly more complex than most. The P_1 antigen is present on the cells of 79% of whites and 94% of African-Americans. When the antigen is not present, the cells are labeled P_2. A characteristic of the P_1 antigen is that it varies in strength on the cells of those that possess it.

The anti-P_1 antibody is a cold-reacting antibody that frequently reacts at temperatures lower than room temperature. If the antibody is suspected, the serum is tested at 17°C. The antibody is an IgM immunoglobulin (see Table 5.3).

Ii ANTIGENS AND ANTIBODIES

The system consists of two antigens that are both present in all individuals (with very, very rare exceptions) in varying amounts. The I antigen is present in large quantities in all adults, whereas the i is present in very small amounts. In contrast, large quantities of i are present on the cells taken from the umbilical cord, and the I antigen is virtually absent. Antibodies to either antigen react best at temper-

EXERCISE 25 CREATING A GENOTYPE

When antibody screening and identification are performed, commercially prepared cells are used. These cells are group O human cells that have been typed for the major blood group systems. When the antibody screening or identification is performed, the patient's serum is reacted with these cells in varying temperatures and media. The reactions are recorded and interpretations made.

When the cells are provided by the manufacturer, the antigen types are provided in an enclosure known as antigram (see Unit 6). This antigram is used after the serum has reacted with the cells to determine the specificity of the antibody. Sample antigrams will be used in this exercise to aid in the understanding of genotype and the scope of antigens present on an individual red blood cell.

This exercise may be performed by each student or in small groups. The instructor will provide antigrams from cell identification panels to each student or group. Using this antigram, each student or group should:

1. With the assistance of the instructor, examine the antigram for an understanding of the "layout" of the cell typings.
2. Examine one cell on the antigram and determine whether that cell is positive or negative for each of the antigens discussed in the previous section.
3. Explain your determination to either the instructor or a partner.
4. With the guidance of the instructor, create a genotype of the antigram cell considering Lewis, P, and MNSs blood group systems.

atures colder than room temperature and are not frequently seen in routine testing for that reason. Anti-i is frequently seen in the serum of persons who have recently experienced infectious mononucleosis.

TESTING FOR ANTIGENS WITH COLD-REACTING ANTISERA

Each antigen discussed will react with specific antisera. These antisera are either human products or lectins that may be purchased commercially. The manufacturer provides a package insert with each antisera. Each antisera should be tested with both a positive and a negative control each day of use.

SYSTEMS WITH WARM-REACTING ANTIBODIES

The previous sections described antibodies that tend to react at cold temperatures. These systems did include some examples that were a part of a cold-reacting group but tended to react in warm temperatures at the anti-human globulin phase such as "s." Bearing this in mind, this division of antigen-antibody systems by reaction temperatures is a loose classification.

The antibodies that react at warm temperatures are reactive at 37°C and most often react at the anti-human globulin phase of testing. They include antibodies that are considered clinically significant and most likely to cause both hemolytic disease of the newborn and hemolytic transfusion reaction.

EXERCISE 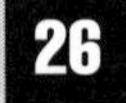

TESTING FOR ANTIGENS WITH COLD-REACTING ANTISERA

The instructor will provide available antisera that may be tested at room temperature and an anticoagulated or clotted blood sample. The students should work individually or in small groups to complete the following:

1. Choose one or more antisera to test with the blood sample provided by the instructor.
2. Read the package insert for the antisera(s).
3. Prepare a worksheet with the help of the instructor.
4. Wearing gloves and goggles, prepare a 5% cell suspension of the blood sample.
5. Test the sample provided with each antisera as indicated in the package insert.
6. In parallel with the patient sample, test positive and negative controls.
7. Record results on worksheet.
8. Repeat steps 5 through 7 with additional antiseras, if possible.
9. Dispose of all waste in a puncture-proof biohazard container.

KELL BLOOD GROUP SYSTEM

The two principal antigens in this blood group system are K (Kell) and k (cellano). These antigens are alleles and are inherited in a Mendelian fashion. The possible genotypes for an individual are *KK*, *Kk*, and *kk*. The k antigen is a high-incidence antigen present in approximately 98% of the white population. Therefore, the *KK* genotype is rare. The frequency of both antigens is summarized in Table 5.2.

There are two additional loci where genes belonging to the Kell system are found. At one locus are the alleles Kp^a and Kp^b; Js^a and Js^b are a second set of alleles at another locus. Each set of alleles is inherited in the Mendelian fashion with three possible sets of genotypes.

Kell Blood Group Antibodies

Antibodies to the K and k antigens are summarized in Table 5.4. These antibodies are primarily IgG antibodies optimally reactive at 37°C in anti-human globulin phase of testing. Both antibodies are capable of causing hemolytic disease of the newborn as well as hemolytic transfusion reaction.

KIDD BLOOD GROUP ANTIGENS

Within the Kidd blood group, there are two primary antigens that are alleles. These antigens are Jk^a and Jk^b (pronounced by saying each letter: "J K A"). These two alleles are inherited in the Mendelian fashion. Three possible genotypes exist. These are Jk^aJk^a, Jk^aJk^b, Jk^bJk^b. The frequencies of these antigens are summarized in Table 5.2.

Kidd Blood Group Antibodies

These antibodies are stimulated by direct exposure via either pregnancy or transfusion. They are typically IgG, anti-human globulin–reactive antibodies. Characteristics of these antibodies are summarized in Table 5.4.

These antibodies have several characteristics that make them known as the "treacherous Kidds." The antigens are not very antigenic and do not stimulate a very strong antibody response. Therefore, the antibodies are often not very strong. In addition, they tend to decrease in strength in the patient's serum with the passage of time. They will sometimes decrease in strength **(titer)** to a point where they cannot be detected with testing. If, inadvertently, the patient receives the antigen in a transfusion, the antibody will be restimulated in a secondary reaction and cause what is known as a "delayed transfusion reaction." This will be discussed further in Unit 8.

The fact that Kidd antibodies decrease in strength is important for the laboratory worker. These antibodies will also display dosage, and the weakened antibody will react more strongly with cells that possess a stronger antigen. The test results should be carefully evaluated if potential for a Kidd antibody exists.

DUFFY BLOOD GROUP ANTIGENS

The Duffy blood group system consists of many antigens. The principal two antigens to be considered here are the alleles Fy^a and Fy^b (pronounced "Duffy a" and "Duffy b"). These antigens are inherited in the same fashion as other systems discussed and three genotypes are possible: Fy^aFy^a, Fy^aFy^b, Fy^bFy^b. The frequencies are summarized in Table 5.2.

Antibodies to Duffy Blood Group

These antibodies are characteristically IgG, anti-human globulin–reactive antibodies that have been actively stimulated through direct antigen exposure. The antibodies are capable of causing hemolytic disease of the newborn and hemolytic transfusion reaction. Characteristics of these antibodies are summarized in Table 5.4.

Testing for Antigens in Blood Group Systems with Warm-Reacting Antibodies

As with all antigen testing discussed, testing for the antigens on the surface of the cell involves the use of a specific antisera that contains an antibody specific for the antigen. The antisera may be obtained from a commercial manufacturer. They are of human origin and should be treated as a potential biohazard.

When performing these antigen typings, the antisera will most often be reactive at the anti-human globulin phase of testing. Red cells and antisera will be incubated at 37°C, washed three or four times after incubation. Anti-human globulin sera is then added. For a description of this method see Unit 2.

EXERCISE 27 CREATING A GENOTYPE

This exercise may be performed by each student or in small groups. The instructor will provide antigrams from cell identification panels to each student or group. Using this antigram, each student or group should:

1. Examine one cell on the antigram and determine whether that cell is positive or negative for each of the antigens discussed in the previous sections on warm-reactive antibodies.
2. Explain your determination to either the instructor or a partner.
3. Create a genotype for the antigram cell considering Kell, Kidd, and Duffy blood group systems.

EXERCISE 28 TESTING RED BLOOD CELLS FOR ANTIGENS WITH WARM-REACTING ANTISERA

The instructor will provide available antisera and an anticoagulated or clotted blood sample to be tested at 37°C and with AHG sera. The students should work individually or in small groups to complete the following:

1. Choose one or more antisera to test with the blood sample provided by the instructor.
2. Read the package insert for the antisera(s).
3. Prepare a worksheet with the help of the instructor.
4. Wearing gloves and goggles, prepare a 5% cell suspension of the blood sample.
5. Test the sample provided with the antisera as indicated in the package insert.
6. In parallel with the patient sample, test positive and negative controls.
7. Record results on worksheet.
8. Repeat steps 5 through 7 with additional antiseras if possible.
9. Dispose of all biohazardous waste in a puncture-proof container.

SUMMARY

Red blood cells have a variety of surface antigens. These antigens are present in different combinations in each individual. With few exceptions, the antigens are inherited in a Mendelian fashion and are expressed in a codominant fashion. These antigens, when not genetically present, may serve as immunogens and stimulate that individual to respond by producing an antibody. The antibodies are significant if they react at warm (body) temperatures and particularly at the antihuman globulin phase. Cold-reacting antibodies present interference in testing; however, they are most often not clinically significant nor will they be incriminated in reactions to transfusion.

Specific antigen systems can be loosely divided into those that have antibodies that are reactive at cold temperatures and those that are warm reacting. The systems with cold-reacting antibodies include Ii, P, MN, and Lewis. Those with warm-reacting antibodies include the Kell, Kidd, and Duffy systems. The Rh system would also be included in the category with warm-reacting antibodies.

The technician must understand the existence of these antigens and the potential for the antibodies to be present. Unit 6 will discuss how the technician will detect and identify these unexpected antibodies in the patient's serum.

REVIEW QUESTIONS

1. Antigen system *not* initially present on red blood cell surface is
   a. Duffy
   b. Lewis
   c. MNSs
   d. P
2. Universal antigen is found on the cells of
   a. no persons
   b. very few persons
   c. approximately half of all persons
   d. the majority of persons
3. I antigen is found in
   a. all newborns; no adults
   b. no newborns; all adults
   c. no human beings
   d. all persons to some degree
4. When testing for any antigen, the antibody used most often comes from a
   a. goat
   b. human
   c. mouse
   d. rabbit
5. A high-incidence antigen is present in
   a. no persons
   b. very low percentages
   c. different amounts on each persons cells
   d. a large percentage of individuals
6. An antibody that reacts best at temperatures less than body temperatures is
   a. anti-I
   b. anti-K
   c. anti-k
   d. anti-s
7. The U antigen is present as a (an)
   a. low-frequency antigen
   b. infrequently encountered antigen
   c. universal antigen
   d. antigen found only at 17°C or less
8. Infectious mononucleosis occurs with the result being a serum antibody that may appear like
   a. anti-Le^a
   b. anti-I
   c. anti-i
   d. anti-P_1

9. Frequencies of antigens in white and African-American populations are
   a. always the same
   b. sometimes the same
   c. never the same
   d. always within 2 percentage points
10. The P_2 phenotype is that present when
   a. P_1 is present in the homozygous state
   b. P_1 is completely absent
   c. P_1 antigen is very weak
   d. P_2 antigen is present in a homozygous state

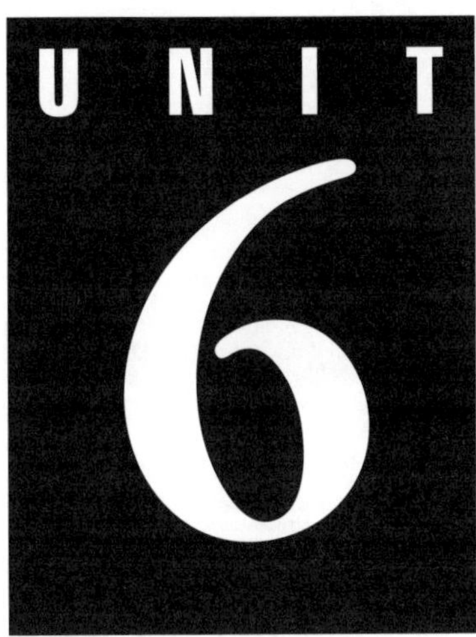

Testing for Unexpected Antibodies

LEARNING OBJECTIVES

After studying this unit, it is the responsibility of the student to know the following objectives:

- **Define terms listed in the glossary.**
- **Describe the principles behind the indirect and direct antiglobulin tests.**
- **Apply the principles of indirect antiglobulin tests to specific test methods.**
- **Perform antibody screen, antibody identification, and direct antiglobulin tests.**

GLOSSARY

antibody identification test performed using a panel of red cells with known antigen content; used to identify the specific antibody or combination of antibodies in the fluid being tested.

antibody screen test performed by mixing patient or donor serum with cells of known antigen content to detect the presence of atypical antibodies.

antigram chart describing the antigen content of the cells used for antibody screen or antibody identification tests.

atypical antibodies antibodies found either in the serum or on the cells that are unanticipated or not found under normal circumstances.

direct antiglobulin test (DAT) test that detects the presence of antibody on the surface of red cells.

eluate liquid harvested after an elution is performed.

elution method used to remove antibodies from the surface of red cells for testing purposes.

low ionic strength saline (LISS) enhancement media.

panel series of cells from different donors used in the antibody identification test.

parallel testing series of tests performed under identical conditions to the patient or control tests; used to rule out contamination or other interferences.

polyethylene glycol (PEG) enhancement media.

proteolytic enzymes enzymes that serve to break down proteins.

INTRODUCTION

To follow the information presented in the previous units, it is important to present methods for the detection and identification of antibodies outlined in Units 4 and 5. This is important for transfusion safety and diagnosis of clinical conditions. This unit will put into perspective those antibodies previously discussed. The division of antibody identification falls into two broad categories: those found on red cells and those present in serum. A logical progression of antibody detection to specific identification will be outlined. The test methods incorporate the anti-human globulin test outlined in Unit 2.

ANTIBODY DETECTION

With the exception of ABO antibodies, the presence of antibodies either in the serum or on the surface of the red cells is an unexpected finding in the blood bank. It is, however, a situation that may influence the successful outcome of a transfusion. Recall that under most circumstances antibodies are developed only if the antigens are not present on an individual's red cells, as stated by Landsteiner's law. Antigens discussed in Units 4 and 5 may stimulate antibody production after exposure in an antigen-negative individual.

Along with ABO and Rh testing, a test performed in the blood bank to detect antibodies in the serum is the **antibody screen** test (sometimes referred to as the anti-human globulin test). This test detects antibodies directed against red cell antigens but found in the serum. If this test is positive and antibodies are present in the serum, a more definitive test known as an **antibody identification** or **panel** is performed. For both antibody screen and identification tests, a sample collected in a plain red-top tube is the ideal specimen. Anticoagulated specimens and specimens collected in tubes with serum separators are not acceptable. As with any other blood bank test, proper patient identification, as determined by the institution, is imperative.

A second test performed to detect antibodies is the **direct antiglobulin test (DAT).** It is a test that detects antibodies coating the surface of the red blood cells *in vivo*. These antibodies are also identified by using an antibody identification or panel. This identification can only be accomplished after the antibodies have been removed from the cells by a process known as **elution**. For a summary of antibody-detection techniques and the methods of testing that lead to the identification of these antibodies, refer to the flow chart in Figure 6.1.

DETECTION OF ANTIBODIES IN SERUM

Patient and donor serum is screened for **atypical antibodies,** using commercially prepared cells. These cells are human products and present a potential biohazard to the user. They are group O cells that have been tested for the presence of the most commonly encountered antigens. This provides a product that has known antigen content. The cells are provided from the manufacturer in sets of

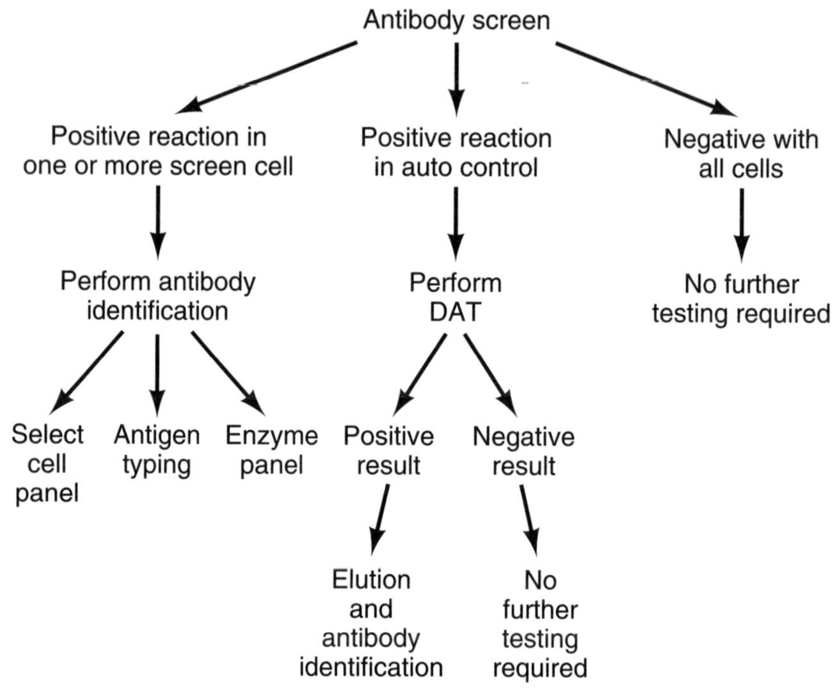

fig. 6.1. Flow chart for antibody identification.

either two or three vials. Each vial contains cells from a single, different donor. The vials are provided with a description of the antigen content of each of the cells. This description is provided in a chart known as an **antigram**. See Figure 6.2 for a sample antigram.

When the test is performed, each vial of cells is tested with the serum of the patient or donor. The test is performed including different conditions of reactivity with variation in the temperature and media of reactivity. The media of reactivity include saline, albumin, **low ionic strength saline (LISS)**, **polyethylene glycol (PEG),** and AHG sera. Reaction media used are chosen at the discretion of the institution.

Results from each phase are recorded and evaluated at the end of the testing. Since this is a screening test, the results indicate the presence of an antibody, but not the specific antibody. By using the antigrams and knowing the temperature and media of reactivity of the potential antibodies, the possibilities may be narrowed, but a more definitive diagnosis is provided by the use of the antibody identification panel.

	D	C	E	$\bar{c}$	$\bar{e}$	K	k	Fy^a	Fy^b	Jk^a	Jk^b	Le^a	Le^b	S	$\bar{s}$	M	N	P_1
I	+	+	0	0	+	0	+	0	+	+	+	0	+	+	0	+	0	+
II	+	0	+	+	+	+	+	+	+	0	+	0	+	0	+	0	+	0

fig. 6.2. Antigram for an antibody screen.

EXERCISE 29 INTERPRETATION OF ANTIGRAM RESULTS

In small groups, students will evaluate sample antigrams from antibody screen cells that are provided by the instructor. The students should evaluate these antigrams and incorporate knowledge from Unit 5 to answer the following questions.

1. What are the optimal temperature and media for the antibody?
2. With which screening cells does the antibody react?
3. List potential antibodies, using all information given.
4. The instructor should check the work.

EXERCISE 30 ANTIBODY SCREEN TEST

This antibody screen procedure may be adapted to antibody screen cells from any manufacturer or using any number of cells.

Equipment:
Gloves
Goggles
10 × 75 or 12 × 75 mm test tubes
0.85% saline in a wash bottle
Laboratory marker
Gauze or laboratory tissues
Antibody screen cells with antigrams
Check cells
LISS (or other enhancement media)
Anti-human globulin sera (AHG)
Transfer pipets
Serological centrifuge
Agglutination viewer
37°C heat block
Test tube rack
Timer
Beaker with disinfectant
Centrifuged clotted blood sample
Worksheet (provided by the instructor or prepared by each student)
Puncture-proof biohazard container

Procedure:

1. Wearing gloves and goggles, prepare a 5% washed cell preparation as described in Exercise 15.

EXERCISE 30 ANTIBODY SCREEN TEST *(continued)*

2. Label one tube for each screening cell to be used and a tube for the autocontrol. Be certain to include proper patient identification on the tubes.
3. Using a transfer pipet, place 2 drops of serum into each of the tubes.
4. Add one drop of *thoroughly mixed* cell suspension from the screening cell vials to each tube as labeled, for example, tube I will receive 1 drop of screen cell I.
5. Add one drop of patient's 5% cell suspension to the autocontrol tube.
6. Mix well and centrifuge for 15 seconds (or the time indicated on the centrifuge).
7. Examine the supernatant for hemolysis as each tube is removed from the centrifuge.
8. Handling one tube at a time, resuspend cells by gently agitating while examining for agglutination with a good light source. An agglutination viewer is ideal.
9. Record results as "Immediate spin saline." Be sure to grade all reactions. Each tube should continue through all phases of testing, even if positive at a previous phase.
10. Add 2 drops of LISS or other enhancement media to each tube. Mix.

NOTE: If an enhancement media other than LISS is used, check manufacturer's instructions prior to use.

11. Incubate all tubes at 37°C for the time designated by the manufacturer for this media. Be sure to set a timer.

NOTE: Incubation time will vary with the enhancement media used. A minimum incubation time for LISS may be 5 minutes. Manufacturer's instructions should be checked for the media being used. Overincubation may cause the antibodies to become dissociated from the antigens on the red cells.

12. When the incubation is complete, centrifuge the tubes for 15 seconds (or the time designated for the centrifuge).
13. Repeat steps 7 and 8.
14. Record results as "LISS." Be sure to grade all reactions. Each tube should continue through all phases of testing, even if positive at a previous phase.
15. Wash the serum/cell mixtures as outlined in Exercise 13.
16. After a total of three or four washes add 2 drops of AHG to each tube.

EXERCISE 30 ANTIBODY SCREEN TEST *(continued)*

17. Mix and centrifuge for 15 seconds (or the time designated on the centrifuge).
18. Repeat steps 7 and 8.

Note: If an agglutination viewer with a magnifying mirror is not available, all negative results should be checked microscopically and the results recorded as "Microscopic."

19. Record results as "AHG." Be sure to grade all reactions. Each tube should continue through all phases of testing, even if positive at a previous phase.
20. To each negative tube add 2 drops of check cells.
21. Centrifuge for 15 seconds.
22. Repeat step 8.
23. Record results as "CC." It is not necessary to grade check cells, but rather indicate as positive or negative. If the check cells do not produce a positive result, the test should be repeated.
24. Interpretation of the results are made as "positive" or "negative." Agglutination at any phase indicates a positive test. Check cell results should disregarded when making interpretation of the test. Positive tests require investigation to determine the etiology of the antibody.
25. Discard all biohazardous waste in a puncture-proof biohazard container.

ANTIBODY IDENTIFICATION

The presence of a positive antibody screen test requires the identification of the antibody present. If the antibody is present in the serum and the antibody screen cells present with a positive result, then an antibody identification panel is necessary. If only the autocontrol is positive, a direct antiglobulin test is necessary.

A panel is a series of red cells from different donors that have been antigen typed for the common red cell antigens. These cells are all from group O donors and are potentially biohazardous. The panel may consist of any number of cells, but most commonly there are between eight and sixteen different cells included in the panel.

A panel is tested in the same manner as an antibody screen. The patient's serum constitutes the unknown with the potential for presence of antibody, whereas the cells represent known antigens. Varying temperatures and media are used to encourage the antigen-antibody reaction. Results are interpreted and either provide a definitive identification or indicate that further testing is necessary.

EXERCISE 31

EXAMINATION OF ANTIBODY IDENTIFICATION PANEL SHEETS

Antigram sheets are provided with each panel that is commercially prepared. Each student should examine a blank antibody identification sheet and observe the items outlined below.

1. The lot number of the panel in use is present on each sheet provided with the panel. Locate this lot number on the panel sheet.

NOTE: It is imperative that the sheet being used correspond to the lot number on the panel. Otherwise the results obtained will not provide a pattern useful for distinguishing the antibody or antibodies present.

2. Patient identification section. Pertinent patient information is recorded here.
3. Results section. A location to record the interpretation of antibody or antibodies identified.
4. Patient cell typings are recorded in the blank space at the bottom of each antigen column. The patient may not be typed for all of these antigens in the testing process.
5. ABO testing results. These test results may be copied from a previous worksheet.
6. DAT results. DAT results may provide insight into the proper identification of antibodies that are reacting with antigens on the patient cells.
7. It is appropriate that all of these sections be completed to give the technician a broad view of all of the test results condensed onto one page.

EXERCISE 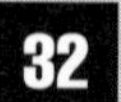

ANTIBODY IDENTIFICATION PANEL

The antibody identification panel provides a series of cells to react with serum suspected of containing an antibody directed against one of the common red cell antigens.

Equipment:
Gloves
Goggles
10 × 75 or 12 × 75 mm test tubes
0.85% saline in a wash bottle

EXERCISE 32 ANTIBODY IDENTIFICATION PANEL *(continued)*

Laboratory marker
Gauze or laboratory tissues
Antibody identification panel with antigram
Check cells
LISS (or other enhancement media)
Anti-human globulin sera (AHG)
Transfer pipets
Serological centrifuge
Agglutination viewer
37°C heat block
Test tube rack
Timer
Beaker with disinfectant
Centrifuged clotted blood sample
Antigram that accompanies the panel
Puncture-proof biohazard container

Procedure:

1. Complete all available information on the antigram.
2. Wearing gloves and goggles, prepare a 5% washed cell suspension of the patient's cells, as described in Exercise 13.
3. Label one tube for each panel cell to be used and a tube for the autocontrol. Be certain to include proper patient identification on the tubes.
4. Using a transfer pipet, place 2 drops of serum into each of the tubes.
5. Add one drop of *thoroughly mixed* cell suspension from the panel cell vials to each tube as labeled, for example, tube 1 will receive 1 drop of panel cell 1.

NOTE: Be sure to read the labels.

6. Add one drop of patient's 5% cell suspension to the autocontrol tube.
7. Mix well and centrifuge for 15 seconds (or the time indicated on the centrifuge).
8. Examine the supernatant for hemolysis as each tube is removed from the centrifuge.
9. Handling one tube at a time, resuspend cells by gently agitating while examining for agglutination with a good light source. An agglutination viewer is ideal.
10. Record results into the first column of the antigram as "Immediate spin saline." Be sure to grade all reactions. Each tube should continue through all phases of testing, even if positive at a previous phase.

EXERCISE 32 ANTIBODY IDENTIFICATION PANEL *(continued)*

11. Add 2 drops of LISS to each tube. Mix. (Another enhancement media may be used.)
12. Incubate all tube at 37°C for the time recommended by the manufacturer of the enhancement media minutes. Be sure to set a timer.

Note: Incubation time will vary with the enhancement media used. Be certain to read the manufacturer's directions included with the product. Overincubation may cause the antibodies to become dissociated from the antigens on the surface of the red cell.

13. When the incubation is complete, centrifuge the tubes for 15 seconds (or the time designated for the centrifuge).
14. Repeat steps 8 and 9.
15. Record results as "LISS." Be sure to grade all reactions. All tubes should continue through all phases of testing, even if positive at a previous phase.
16. Wash the serum/cell mixtures, as outlined in Exercise 13.
17. After a total of three or four washes, add 2 drops of AHG to each tube.
18. Repeat steps 8 and 9.

Note: If an agglutination viewer with a magnifying mirror is not available, all negative results should be checked microscopically. The results should then be recorded as "Microscopic."

19. Record results as "AHG." Be sure to grade all reactions. Each tube should continue through all phases of testing, even if positive at a previous phase.
20. To each negative tube add 2 drops of check cells.
21. Repeat steps 8 and 9.
22. Record results as "CC." It is not necessary to grade check cells, but rather indicate as positive or negative. If check cells in any tube do not have a positive reaction, the test must be repeated.

See Figure 6.3 for an example of a completed panel sheet.

23. Interpretation of the results is made using the method described in Exercise 33. If a definitive identification cannot be made, further testing will be required. Disregard check cell reactions when interpreting the results for the test.
24. Discard all biohazardous waste in a puncture-proof biohazard container.

Cell No.	D	C	E	c	e	f	K	k	Fy^a	Fy^b	Jk^a	Jk^b	Xg^a	Le^a	Le^b	S	s	M	N	P_1	IS	37°	AHG	C.C.
1	+	+	0	0	+	0	0	+	+	+	+	0	+	0	+	+	+	+	0	0	0	1+	2+	
2	+	+	0	0	+	0	+	+	+	$+^{w}$	+	+	+	0	+	+	+	+	0	0	0	1+	2+	+
3	+	0	+	+	0	0	0	+	+	0	0	+	+	0	+	0	+	0	+	$+^{s}$	0	0	0	+
4	+	0	0	+	+	+	0	+	0	0	+	+	+	0	0	0	+	+	+	$+^{s}$	0	0	0	
5	0	+	0	+	+	+	0	+	0	+	+	+	0	0	+	+	0	+	0	+	0	1+	2+	+
6	0	0	+	+	+	+	0	+	0	+	+	+	+	0	+	0	+	+	0	+	0	0	0	+
7	0	0	0	+	+	+	+	+	0	+	0	+	+	0	+	0	+	+	+	0	0	0	0	+
8	0	0	0	+	+	+	+	+	+	0	+	0	+	0	0	+	+	+	+	0	0	0	0	+
9	0	0	0	+	+	+	0	+	+	0	+	0	+	+	0	+	0	+	0	$+^{w}$	0	0	0	+
10	0	0	0	+	+	+	0	+	0	+	0	+	+	+	0	0	+	0	+	+	0	0	0	+
11														0	0						0	0	0	+

(IS, 37°, AHG and C.C. columns are grouped under the header "Test Results".)

fig. 6.3. Example of a completed panel sheet.

Interpretation of the antibody identification panel is done using an elimination method. Elimination is a systematic procedure. It uses the cells with no reactivity at any phase to eliminate potential antibodies to antigens present on that cell. The method is useful but not foolproof. Antibodies to antigens that display dosage or combinations of antibodies will present a challenge and may not provide a definitive resolution using the elimination method.

E X E R C I S E 

EXERCISE 33 ELIMINATION METHOD TO INTERPRET ANTIBODY IDENTIFICATION PANELS

For this exercise, students may use results from panels tested in Exercise 32 or completed antigrams provided by the instructor.

Equipment:
Completed antigrams
Ruler
Pencil

1. Place the antigram on a flat surface and examine the results column. Do not consider the check cell results.
2. Determine the first cell that elicited no response when reacted with the serum.
3. Place a straightedge under the cell typings and results for that cell (see Figure 6.4).
4. Examine the typing results for that cell. For each antigen that typed positive on that cell, place a line through that antigen designation on the top of the page (see Figure 6.4).
5. Repeat this with each cell that produced no reaction, until all of the cells have been considered.
6. Antigens not crossed with a line are those that have not been eliminated as corresponding to possible antibodies in the serum.
7. The pattern of cell reactions is examined and compared to the vertical pattern of reactivity for each antigen. If an exact match is found, this is most likely the antibody present. It is ideal to rule out all other possible antibodies, since a combination of more than one antibody is possible (see Figure 6.5).
8. If an exact pattern of reactivity is not seen, other test methods are used to determine the antibody or antibodies present. These techniques will be discussed in the following sections.
9. As you examine the patterns of reactivity for each antigen, note that some antigens are not found on any of the cells in the panel. For these antigens, it is impossible to rule them out using the elimination system. Whereas it is not correct to say that antibodies directed against those antigens are not present, it is impossible to rule them out with a panel that does not have the antigen present.

EXERCISE 33 ELIMINATION METHOD TO INTERPRET ANTIBODY IDENTIFICATION PANELS *(continued)*

10. Examine the pattern of reactivity on the antigram and determine if there is an exact match of patterns. If not, identify all possible antibodies.
11. List the possible antibodies in the place on the antigram that is designated for this purpose. The proper way to list them is as "anti-C" or using the Greek letter alpha followed by the antibody, for example, "α-C." This is an example of a potential antibody identification result.
12. The instructor should check the results obtained.
13. All steps are repeated with each antigram to be interpreted.

When the results of the antibody identification are not definitive, further testing may be done to narrow the possibilities. This further testing includes altering reaction temperatures, enzyme testing, antigen typing, select cell panels, cold panels, and absorption. Enzyme testing will be discussed in this section. Antigen typing was discussed in Unit 5. The more inquisitive student is referred to a text on immunohematology for a discussion of select cell panels and absorption.

ENZYME TESTING

Enzymes are used in blood bank testing to aid in identification of antibodies. **Proteolytic enzymes**, such as ficin and papain, affect antigen-antibody reactions in two ways. They either enhance the reaction and make it stronger or inhibit it and result in no reaction. When the reactions are inhibited, it is due to the destruction of antigens on the surface of the cells. Some antigens are enhanced or made more readily available by enzymes. (See Table 6.1 for a summary of the effects of enzymes.) Because they destroy the reactions of some antibodies, the use of enzymes may help to identify antibodies in combination in a serum. Be careful, however, not to exclusively use enzyme panels, since some potentially dangerous antibodies may be missed.

Table 6.1. Effects of Enzymes on Antigens

Antigens Enhanced by Enzymes	Antigens Destroyed by Enzymes
Rh	Duffy
Kidd	MN
I	
Lewis	
P_1	

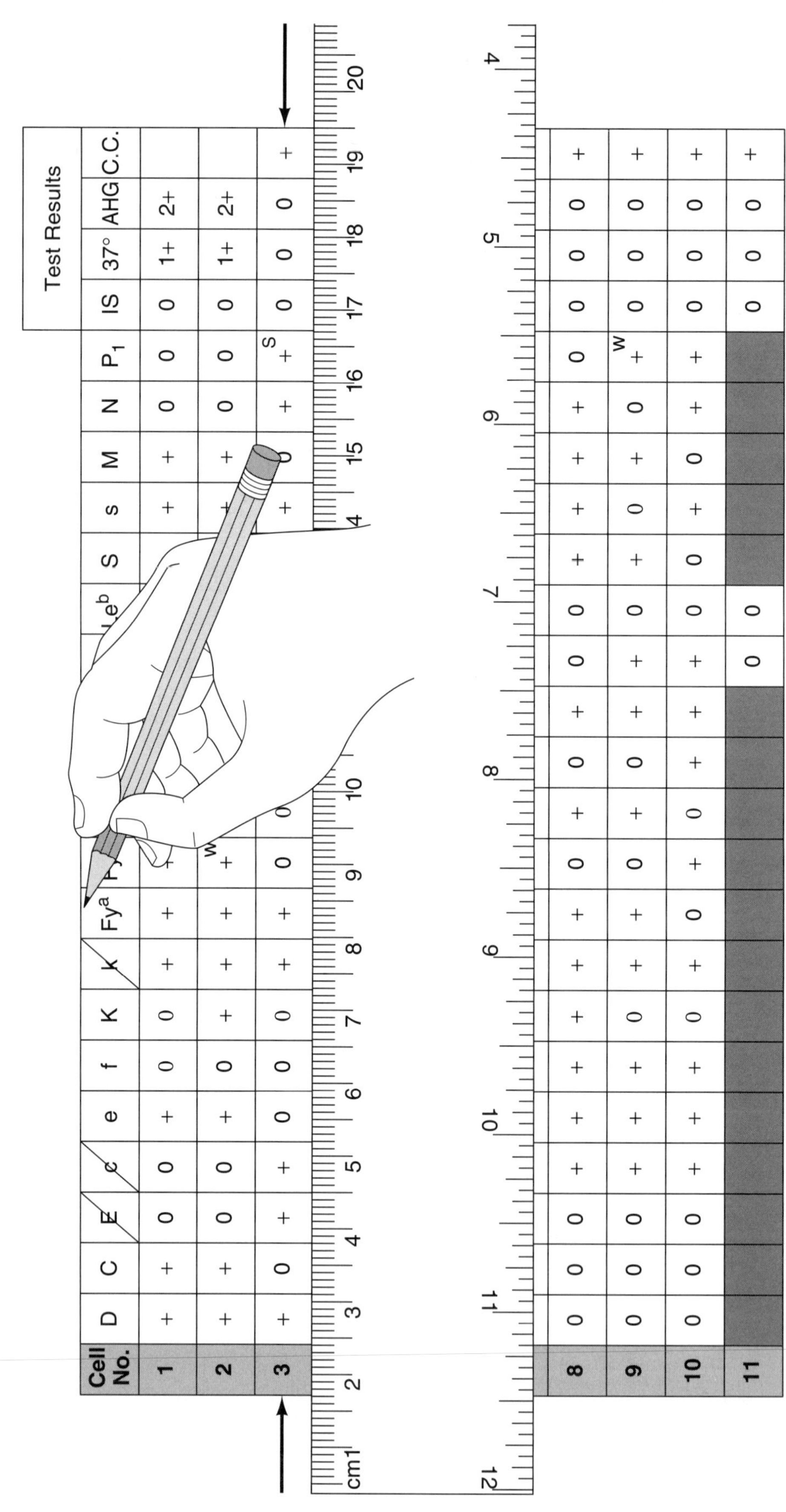

fig. 6.4. Panel interpretation using the elimination system with a straightedge.

Cell No.	D	C	E	c	e	f	K	k	Fy^a	Fy^b	Jk^a	Jk^b	Xg^a	Le^a	Le^b	S	s	M	N	P_1	IS	37°	AHG	C.C.
1	+	+	0	0	+	0	0	+	+	+	+	0	+	0	+	+	+	+	0	0	0	1+	2+	
2	+	+	0	0	+	0	+	+	+	+w	+	+	+	0	+	+	+	+	0	0	0	1+	2+	
3	+	0	+	+	0	0	0	+	+	0	0	+	+	0	+	0	+	0	+	+s	0	0	0	+
4	+	0	0	+	+	+	0	+	0	0	+	+	+	0	0	0	+	+	+	+s	0	0	0	+
5	0	+	0	+	+	+	0	+	0	+	+	+	0	0	+	+	0	+	0	+	0	1+	2+	
6	0	0	+	+	+	+	0	+	0	+	+	+	+	0	+	0	+	+	0	+	0	0	0	+
7	0	0	0	+	+	+	+	+	0	+	0	+	+	0	+	0	+	+	+	0	0	0	0	+
8	0	0	0	+	+	+	+	+	+	0	+	0	+	0	0	+	+	+	+	0	0	0	0	+
9	0	0	0	+	+	+	0	+	+	0	+	0	+	+	0	+	0	+	0	+w	0	0	0	+
10	0	0	0	+	+	+	0	+	0	+	0	+	+	+	0	0	+	0	+	+	0	0	0	+
11														0	0						0	0	0	+

Interpretation: Anti-C

fig. 6.5. Completed panel interpretation.

Enzymes may be used in blood bank testing in two ways. Cells may be treated and the excess enzyme washed away. This is the indirect method. The direct method involves adding enzyme to the serum/cell test mixture in much the same manner that albumin or other enhancement media are added. The indirect method is more sensitive and provides a stronger effect but is more time consuming.

EXERCISE  ENZYME TREATMENT OF RED BLOOD CELLS

This exercise may be performed individually or in small groups or reviewed if the procedure is impractical for the situation.

Equipment:
Goggles
Gloves
10 × 75 or 12 × 75 mm test tubes
Panel cells
Enzyme prepared and ready for use
Transfer pipet
0.85% saline in a wash bottle
Gauze or laboratory tissues
Laboratory marker
Beaker with disinfectant
37°C heat block
Serological centrifuge
Puncture-proof biohazard container

Procedure:
1. Label a tube for each cell in the panel.
2. Wearing gloves and goggles, place 1 drop of cells into each tube as labeled.
3. Add 1 drop of the prepared enzyme solution to each tube.
4. Incubate at 37°C for 10 minutes.

Note: Do not overincubate.

5. Wash all tubes with saline three or four times, as described in Exercise 13.
6. Blot dry with gauze or lab tissues on the last wash.
7. Testing may proceed as indicated in the antibody identification panel procedure. The primary difference is that no albumin or enhancement media are added. The enzyme serves as the enhancement media.
8. See Figure 6.6 for examples of antibody identification panels that were enhanced or destroyed by enzymes.

Cell No.	D	C	E	c	e	f	K	k	Fy^a	Fy^b	Jk^a	Jk^b	Xg^a	Le^a	Le^b	S	s	M	N	P_1	Test Results IS	Test Results 37°	Test Results AHG	Test Results C.C.	Enzyme Test Results IS	Enzyme Test Results 37°	Enzyme Test Results AHG	Enzyme Test Results C.C.
1	+	+	0	0	+	0	0	+	+	+	+	0	+	0	+	+	+	+	0	0	0	1+	2+		0	3+	4+	
2	+	+	0	0	+	0	+	+	+	+w	+	+	+	0	+	+	+	+	0	0	0	0	2+		0	3+	4+	
3	+	0	+	+	0	0	0	+	+	0	0	+	+	0	+	0	+	0	+	+s	0	0	0	+	0	0	0	+
4	+	0	0	+	+	+	0	+	0	0	+	+	+	0	0	0	+	+	+	+s	0	0	0	+	0	0	0	+
5	0	+	0	+	+	+	0	+	0	+	+	+	0	0	+	+	0	+	0	+	0	1+	2+		0	3+	4+	
6	0	0	+	+	+	+	0	+	0	+	+	+	+	0	+	0	+	+	0	+	0	0	0	+	0	0	0	+
7	0	0	0	+	+	+	+	+	0	+	0	+	+	0	+	0	+	+	+	0	0	0	0	+	0	0	0	+
8	0	0	0	+	+	+	+	+	+	0	+	0	+	0	0	+	+	+	+	0	0	0	0	+	0	0	0	+
9	0	0	0	+	+	+	0	+	+	0	+	0	+	+	0	+	0	+	0	+w	0	0	0	+	0	0	0	+
10	0	0	0	+	+	+	0	+	0	+	0	+	+	+	0	0	+	0	+	+	0	0	0	+	0	0	0	+
11														0	0						0		0	+	0	0	0	+

fig. 6.6a. Sample panel showing antibody that is enhanced by enzymes.

Cell No.	D	C	E	c	e	f	K	k	Fy^a	Fy^b	Jk^a	Jk^b	Xg^a	Le^a	Le^b	S	s	M	N	P1	Test Results IS	Test Results 37°	Test Results AHG	Test Results C.C.	Enzyme Test Results IS	Enzyme Test Results 37°	Enzyme Test Results AHG	Enzyme Test Results C.C.
1	+	+	0	0	+	0	0	+	+	+	+	0	+	0	+	+	+	+	0	0	0	0	1+		0	0	0	+
2	+	+	0	0	+	0	+	+	+	+w	+	+	+	0	+	+	+	+	0	0	0	0	1+		0	0	0	+
3	+	0	+	+	0	0	0	+	+	0	0	+	+	0	+	0	+	0	+	+s	0	0	1+		0	0	0	+
4	+	0	0	+	+	+	0	+	0	0	+	+	+	0	0	0	+	+	+	+s	0	0	0	+	0	0	0	+
5	0	+	0	+	+	+	0	+	0	+	+	+	0	0	+	+	0	+	0	+	0	0	0	+	0	0	0	+
6	0	0	+	+	+	+	0	+	0	+	+	+	+	0	+	0	+	+	0	+	0	0	0	+	0	0	0	+
7	0	0	0	+	+	+	+	+	0	+	0	+	+	0	+	0	+	+	+	0	0	0	0	+	0	0	0	+
8	0	0	0	+	+	+	+	+	+	0	+	0	+	0	0	+	+	+	+	0	0	0	1+		0	0	0	+
9	0	0	0	+	+	+	0	+	+	0	+	0	+	+	0	+	0	+	0	+w	0	0	1+		0	0	0	+
10	0	0	0	+	+	+	0	+	0	+	0	+	+	+	0	0	+	0	+	+	0	0	0	+	0	0	0	+
11														0	0						0	0	0	+	0	0	0	+

fig. 6.6b. Sample panel showing antibody that is destroyed by enzymes.

EXERCISE 35 INTERPRETATION OF PANELS USING ENZYME TREATED CELLS

Each student should interpret sample panel sheets provided by the instructor. Careful attention should be paid to antibodies that are enhanced or destroyed by enzymes. Follow the protocol below when examining each antigram:

1. Examine the original panel and compare the results to the enzyme panel.
2. Determine if one or more antibodies has been enhanced or destroyed.
3. Check each antibody that was enhanced or destroyed on the list of possible antibodies and try to achieve a match.
4. Discuss the results with a fellow student.
5. Have the instructor check the results.

ANTIGEN TYPING

Antigen typing using specific antisera was discussed in Unit 5. If there are antibodies that cannot be ruled out based on the original panel, antigen typing may be helpful. In order for this procedure to be useful, the autocontrol must be negative at all phases of testing. For each antigen that cannot be ruled out, the technician may perform antigen typing. If the antigen is present, then that antibody is not present as an alloantibody. According to Landsteiner's law, individuals develop antibodies to antigens that are not present on their red cells. The results of the antigen typings are recorded on the bottom of the panel sheet where patient cell results are indicated.

DIRECT ANTIGLOBULIN TEST

Direct antiglobulin test (DAT) is used to detect antibody coating of cells *in vivo*. No incubation phase is necessary, as in the indirect test. The test is performed by preparing a 5% suspension of cells. These cells are placed in a tube and washed three times in the same manner as described in Exercise 13. AHG is added to the cells. More than one type of AHG sera may be used to aid in differentiation of the type of immunoglobulins or complement coating the cells. If more than one type is used, a separate tube is necessary for each type of sera used.

DETERMINATION OF CAUSE FOR POSITIVE DAT

Positive DAT tests are caused by antibodies coating the cells *in vivo*. It is not always possible to determine the exact cause of the problem, but some simple laboratory methods may be used to narrow the etiology. The first of these is to perform the test using varying AHG sera. A positive result in polyspecific AHG

EXERCISE 36 DIRECT ANTIGLOBULIN TEST (DAT)

Each student will perform a DAT test.

Equipment:
Gloves
Goggles
10 × 75 or 12 × 75 mm test tubes
0.85% saline in a wash bottle
5% cell suspension
Laboratory marker
Gauze or laboratory tissues
Check cells
Anti-human globulin sera (AHG)
Transfer pipets
Serological centrifuge
Agglutination viewer
Test tube rack
Beaker with disinfectant
Puncture-proof biohazard container

Procedure:

1. Label the appropriate number of tubes with patient identification. One tube is required for each type of AHG sera. This procedure will use only one type of sera.
2. Wearing gloves and goggles, use a transfer pipet to add 1 drop of 5% cell suspension to a single labeled tube.
3. Wash the cells three or four times, using the procedure described in Exercise 13. Be sure to blot dry on the third wash.
4. Add 2 drops of AHG sera to the tube.
5. Centrifuge for 15 seconds or the time indicated on the centrifuge.
6. Examine for hemolysis and agglutination, using a good light source. Record results. Be sure to grade the agglutination.

NOTE: An agglutination viewer with a magnifying mirror is ideal. If an agglutination viewer is not available, the cells should be examined microscopically.

7. Questionable results may be checked microscopically and the results recorded as "Microscopic."
8. Interpret results as "positive" or "negative."
9. Check cells should be added to all negative tubes.
10. Centrifuge for 15 seconds or the time indicated on the centrifuge.
11. Examine for agglutination. Record results.
12. Have the instructor check results.
13. Dispose of all biohazardous waste into a puncture-proof biohazard container.

indicates that there is either an immunoglobulin, complement, or both coating the cells. One may use monospecific antisera such as anti-IgG or anti-C3 to provide a more specific indication of the cause of the positive test.

ELUTION

Elution is used to remove the substance coating the cells and provide the technician with the ability to try to determine specificity. Elution techniques are many and varied. Methods are summarized in Table 6.2. All elution methods use a series of steps that remove the antibody from the cells. These steps begin with a thorough washing of the cells; the last wash is saved. Most of the methods also destroy the red cells. This means that the cells are no longer available for testing.

Once the elution has been completed, the liquid that is harvested is called the **eluate**. The eluate may be then treated like a serum. When the eluate is tested, **parallel testing** of the last wash is done to be certain that the substances detected in the eluate resulted from the elution procedure, not contamination from insufficient washing techniques.

Many elution procedures use chemicals that require special handling and have noxious fumes. There are elution procedures that are simple and require no

EXERCISE 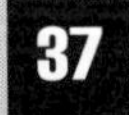

37 DETERMINING ETIOLOGY OF POSITIVE DAT TEST

Each student should consider the following situations and determine a more specific cause of the positive DAT.

Case #1		Case #2		Case #3	
Polyspecific	2+	Polyspecific	1+	Polyspecific	2+
Anti-IgG	2+	Anti-IgG	0	Anti-IgG	1+
Anti-C_3	0	Anti-C_3	1+	Anti-C_3	1+

Students should meet as a group to discuss the outcomes of the assessments with the instructor as a moderator.

Table 6.2. Elution Methods

Heat
Freeze-thaw
Ultrasound
Ether
Digitonin-acid
Cold-acid
Chloroform
Xylene
Methylene chloride

special equipment or chemicals. The type of elution technique used is dependent on the suspected nature of the antibody or the nature of the clinical condition suspected of causing the positive test. Heat and freeze-thaw techniques will be provided in Exercises 38 and 39.

EXERCISE 38 HEAT ELUTION

This technique is useful for evaluating ABO hemolytic disease of the newborn and the removal of IgM antibodies from red blood cells. Students should perform the following procedure either individually or in small groups.

Equipment:
Gloves
Goggles
13 × 100 mm test tubes
0.85% saline in a wash bottle
Centrifuge
Heat block or water bath set at 56°C
Transfer pipets
Laboratory marker
6% bovine albumin (made by diluting 22% or 30% albumin)
Timer
Parafilm
Red cells with a positive DAT test
Puncture-proof biohazard container

Procedure:

1. Label three tubes with patient identification. One tube should then be labeled "washed packed cells," a second labeled "last wash," and a third labeled "eluate."
2. Wearing gloves and goggles, transfer approximately 2 ml of red cells into the test tube labeled "washed packed cells."
3. Wash these cells six times, following Exercise 15.
4. At the end of the last wash, remove the wash saline into the tube labeled "last wash."
5. To the washed packed cells, add an equal volume of 6% albumin. Cover with parafilm. Mix.
6. Place the tube at 56°C for 10 minutes. Set a timer.
7. Invert the tube often during the 10-minute incubation.
8. At the end of 10 minutes, centrifuge the tube for 2 minutes. A heated centrifuge is preferable, but not necessary.
9. Transfer the eluate into the tube labeled "eluate."
10. This eluate may now be tested in the same manner as a serum. Remember to test the last wash in parallel.
11. Discard all biohazardous waste into a puncture-proof biohazard container.

EXERCISE 39 FREEZE-THAW ELUTION (LUI EASY FREEZE ELUTION)

This technique is useful for evaluating ABO hemolytic disease of the newborn. Students should perform the following procedure either individually or in small groups.

Equipment:
Gloves
Goggles
13 × 100 mm test tubes
0.85% saline in a wash bottle
Centrifuge
Freezer set at −20°C to −70°C
Transfer pipets
Laboratory marker
Timer
Parafilm
Red cells with a positive DAT test
Puncture-proof biohazard container

Procedure:

1. Label tubes with patient identification. One tube should be labeled "washed packed cells," a second labeled "last wash," and a third labeled "eluate."
2. Wearing gloves and goggles, transfer approximately 0.5 ml of red cells into the test tube labeled "washed packed cells."

NOTE: Multiple tubes may be required to obtain the volume of eluate required for further testing.

3. Wash these cells six times, following Exercise 15.
4. At the end of the last wash, remove the wash saline into the tube labeled "last wash."
5. To the tube of washed packed cells add 3 drops of saline. Parafilm and mix.
6. Rotate each tube so that the red cell/saline mixture coats the inside of the tube.
7. Place the tube horizontally at −20°C to −70°C for 10 minutes. Set a timer.
8. After 10 minutes, rapidly thaw the tube under warm running water.
9. Centrifuge the tube for 2 minutes.
10. Transfer the supernatant into the tube labeled "eluate."
11. This eluate may now be tested in the same manner as serum. Remember to test the last wash in parallel.
12. Discard all biohazardous waste into a puncture-proof biohazard container.

The most useful testing of an eluate is to perform an antibody identification panel, as is done with serum. If a definitive identification can be made, the causative antibody has been identified. Many times, particularly when the positive DAT is drug related, the antibody cannot be matched to one or more antibodies and is said to be nonspecific.

CLINICAL INDICATIONS OF A POSITIVE DIRECT ANTIGLOBULIN TEST

When the DAT is positive, it indicates that the patient has antibody attached to the red cells that occurred *in vivo*. This may occur in any of a number of autoimmune disorders. It indicates that an autoantibody exists. This antibody is directed against an antigen present on the surface of the patient's red cells and goes against Landsteiner's law. Note also that whenever an autocontrol is positive in the AHG phase of an antibody screen or antibody identification panel, this indicates that an autoantibody may be present. In these cases, the direct antiglobulin test will most likely be positive.

Autoantibodies occur in clinical conditions such as autoimmune hemolytic anemia (AIHA), drug-induced AIHA, hemolytic disease of the newborn (HDN), and hemolytic transfusion reaction (HTR). HDN and HTR will be discussed in later units in this manual.

CAUSES OF FALSE-POSITIVE AND FALSE-NEGATIVE TEST RESULTS FOR ANTI-HUMAN GLOBULIN TESTING

As with any tests, results may be affected by conditions in the test that lend it to being either falsely positive or negative. The potential causes of false positive and negative reactions are summarized in Table 6.3.

Table 6.3. False-Positive and False-Negative Reactions in AHG Testing

False Positives	False Negatives
Interference of cold agglutinating antibodies	Improper interpretation of test results
Interference from intravenous solutions	Not adding sera to the test
Cells from sample collected with a serum separator	Improper incubation time or temperature
Patient allergy to the preservatives in the cell solutions	Improper centrifugation of test
Rouleaux	Inappropriate strength of cell suspensions
Improper interpretation of test results	Outdated cell products
Overcentrifugation	Improper storage of cell products
Inappropriate strength of cell suspension	Contaminated reagents
Contaminated reagents	Not adding reagents
Improper washing	Dilution of AHG sera
	Not washing serum/cell mixture prior to adding AHG sera
	Inadequate washing of cells
	Using cells from a sample collected with an anticoagulant (Indirect test only)

SUMMARY

The detection and identification of antibodies are vital to the daily test performance in the blood bank. The use of the anti-human globulin test methods and their applications is invaluable to the success of proper detection and identification of antibodies as well as determining suitable blood for transfusion. Distinction between the indirect and direct methods is imperative for the technician. The indirect methodology is applied to tests such as antibody screen, antibody identification, antigen typing, and crossmatch. It will be discussed again in Unit 7.

Direct antiglobulin test (DAT) is useful in diagnosis of autoimmune disorders such as autoimmune hemolytic anemia, drug-induced autoimmune hemolytic anemia, hemolytic disease of the newborn, and hemolytic transfusion reaction. Physicians and technicians frequently work together to combine patient history with test results to reach a diagnosis and institute correct treatment for the patient.

The antibody causing the direct antiglobulin test may be removed from the surface of the cells by the procedure known as elution. This eluate may then be used to identify the antibody by applying an antibody identification procedure. Once the antibody is identified, the information may be combined with other data to confirm a diagnosis.

CASE STUDY 5

A 61-year-old male patient was admitted for a laparotomy. Two units of blood were ordered to be crossmatched for possible transfusion. Since no previous records were available for this patient, the technician performed an ABO and Rh and an antibody screen prior to performing the crossmatch. The antibody screen showed positive results and an identification panel was performed. The results of this panel are summarized in Panel A.

QUESTIONS

1. Interpret Panel A. What is the antibody most likely present?
2. If an enzyme panel were performed, what effect would the enzyme have on the reactions of this antibody?
3. What would you expect the results of the patient's antigen typing for the antigen specific to the antibody to be?
4. What steps should the technician take to assure that compatible blood is available for this patient?

	D	C	E	c	e	f	K	k	Fy^a	Fy^b	Jk^a	Jk^b	Xg^a	Le^a	Le^b	S	s	M	N	P_1	Test Results: IS	37°	AHG	C.C.
1	+	+	0	0	+	0	0	+	+	+	+	0	+	0	+	+	+	+	0	0	0	0	1+	
2	+	+	0	0	+	0	+	+	+	$+^w$	+	+	+	0	+	+	+	+	0	0	0	0	1+	
3	+	0	+	+	0	0	0	+	+	0	0	+	+	0	+	0	+	0	+	$+^S$	0	0	0	+
4	+	0	0	+	+	+	0	+	0	0	+	+	+	0	0	0	+	+	+	$+^S$	0	0	1+	
5	0	+	0	+	+	+	0	+	0	+	+	+	0	0	+	+	0	+	0	+	0	0	1+	
6	0	0	+	+	+	+	0	+	0	+	+	+	+	0	+	0	+	+	0	+	0	0	1+	
7	0	0	0	+	+	+	+	+	0	+	0	+	+	0	+	0	+	+	+	0	0	0	0	+
8	0	0	0	+	+	+	+	+	+	0	+	0	+	0	0	+	+	+	+	0	0	0	1+	
9	0	0	0	+	+	+	0	+	+	0	+	0	+	+	0	+	0	+	0	$+^w$	0	0	1+	
10	0	0	0	+	+	+	0	+	0	+	0	+	+	+	0	0	+	0	+	+	0	0	0	+
CORD														0	0						0	0	0	+

Panel A.

CASE STUDY 6

A 72-year-old man admitted for possible bowel obstruction is being prepared for surgery. The surgeon has ordered ABO, Rh, and antibody screen tests, as well as a crossmatch for 2 units of blood. The antibody screen was positive in the autocontrol but not in either of the screening cells.

1. What test would be performed next? What specific reagent(s) would be useful? Why?
2. If the test performed in #1 were positive, what test would be performed next? Why?
3. Since the antibody screen test is negative, is an identification panel on the patient's serum necessary? Why or why not?

REVIEW QUESTIONS

1. The direct anti-globulin test detects
   a. antigen-antibody interactions *in vitro*
   b. antibody attachment to panel cells
   c. antibody attachment *in vivo*
   d. antigen presence on the red cell surface
2. Autoimmune hemolytic anemia is detected using a (an)
   a. antibody screen
   b. direct antiglobulin
   c. antigen typing
   d. panel
3. Indirect enzyme testing involves
   a. use of albumin
   b. adding enzyme to serum/cell mixture
   c. pretreatment of cells
   d. screening cells
4. An antibody screen test is positive. The test that is used to determine a specific antibody is the
   a. DAT
   b. elution
   c. panel
   d. enzyme panel
5. An antibody identification panel is interpreted using a method known as
   a. antigen typing
   b. elution
   c. elimination
   d. pretreatment

6. The last wash from an eluate is used to
   a. reconstitute the red cell suspension
   b. test in parallel
   c. perform a DAT
   d. antigen type
7. Panel cells have been tested for
   a. ABO and Rh antigens only
   b. group O red cell antigens
   c. all red cell antigens that exist
   d. most common red cell antigens
8. Of the following antigens, the one destroyed by enzymes is
   a. Jk^a
   b. P_1
   c. M
   d. I
9. The Lui easy freeze elution is most useful for detecting antibodies to antigens of the
   a. ABO blood group
   b. Rh blood group
   c. I blood group
   d. Kidd blood group
10. If check cells results are negative, the cause may be
    a. inadequate washing of cells
    b. that all cells were properly washed
    c. inadequate tube size
    d. prolonged centrifugation

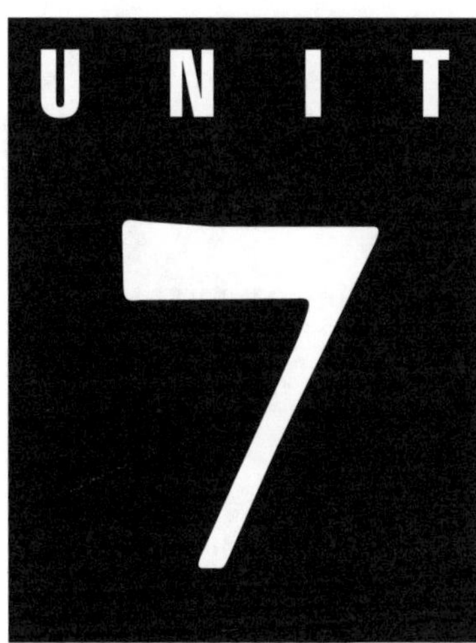

Compatibility Tests, Components, and Donors

LEARNING OBJECTIVES

After studying this unit, it is the responsibility of the student to know the following objectives:

- **Define terms listed in the glossary.**
- **Identify the steps of compatibility testing.**
- **Discuss clerical components of compatibility testing.**
- **Perform compatibility testing at all phases.**
- **List and discuss components available for transfusion.**
- **Outline initial donor testing and tests performed on receipt of blood at remote sites.**

GLOSSARY

anticoagulant chemical substance used to prevent clotting of blood.

compatibility test testing used to determine if blood for transfusion will be safe to transfuse.

compatible serologically nonreactive mixing test.

crossmatch test performed by mixing donor and recipient blood to determine *in vitro* compatibility.

cryoprecipitate concentrated coagulation factor VIII and fibrinogen extracted from fresh frozen plasma.

deglycerolized red cells cells that have been frozen in glycerol, thawed, and washed.

fresh frozen plasma (FFP) plasma extracted and frozen within 6 hours of collection.

frozen thawed red cells cells that have been frozen in glycerol and thawed when ready for transfusion.

immediate spin crossmatch mixing donor and recipient blood and reading for agglutination after the first spin without incubation or enhancement media.

incompatibility reactive when mixed.

leukocyte concentrate white blood cells collected from a single donor by pheresis.

leukocyte poor red cells red cell products prepared by one of several methods to create a product that has a decreased amount of white blood cells.

major crossmatch compatibility test combining recipient's serum with donor's cells.

packed red cells donor unit of red cells from which the plasma has been removed.

pheresis process to remove a portion of whole blood and return the remaining portions of the blood to the donor.

platelet concentrate platelets removed from whole blood and stored for transfusion.

preservative chemical substance that provides substances to prevent deterioration of the cells.

recipient person to receive a transfusion or treatment.

single donor or **liquid plasma** plasma extracted from red cells after the time frame allowable for fresh frozen plasma or plasma with the cryoprecipitate removed; used for volume replacement.

whole blood blood that contains all components.

INTRODUCTION

Compatibility testing is important in the blood bank laboratory. The determination of compatibility of a unit of blood for transfusion is performed each time a transfusion of whole blood or cells is to be given. In combination with compatibility testing, knowledge of donor procedures and components available for transfusion are important for the technician. These three topics will be discussed individually in this unit. Relationships between the topics will be noted.

COMPATIBILITY TESTING

Compatibility testing is a series of procedures designed to ensure the safety of blood for transfusion. *The American Association of Blood Banks (AABB) Technical Manual* and *AABB Standards* outline acceptable procedures for compatibility testing. These guidelines will be discussed in the following sections.

Included in the **compatibility test** is a **crossmatch** that is performed prior to transfusion of **whole blood** or **packed red cells.** The crossmatch combines serum from the **recipient** or patient with cells from the donor. This combination is a **major crossmatch**. Any reaction in the major crossmatch test is considered significant and the cause determined before transfusion of the unit being tested (see Figure 7.1).

MAJOR CROSSMATCH

The major crossmatch is an *in vitro* determination that combines the **recipient**'s serum with a 5% cell suspension of the donor's cells. This test is performed at different phases in the same manner as the antibody screen and antibody identification. The final phase is the anti-human globulin (AHG) test. This is a vital part of the crossmatch. Antibodies that react at the AHG phase are the antibodies that, if present in the recipient, are most likely to cause a reaction *in vivo.*

Historically, a minor crossmatch was done by mixing the serum of the donor with cells from the recipient. The minor crossmatch is no longer performed and will not be discussed further.

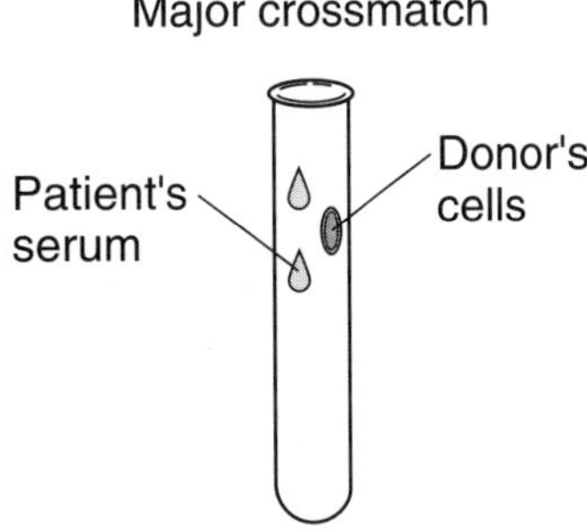

fig. 7.1. Major crossmatch.

The **immediate spin crossmatch** is the first phase of the major crossmatch procedure. This crossmatch mixes recipient's serum with donor's cells. The immediate spin phase is performed and recorded. ABO **incompatibility** will be seen at this phase. Historically, ABO incompatibility has caused most fatal transfusion reactions.

The immediate spin crossmatch for compatibility is performed when the antibody screen has detected no atypical antibodies and no history of clinically significant antibodies is known. The AABB has established that, under these circumstances, the complete crossmatch at all phases is not necessary.

TEST METHODS FOR THE MAJOR CROSSMATCH

The complete crossmatch includes all phases of testing: immediate spin, enhancement media, AHG, and check cells. Requirements for compatibility testing vary by accrediting agency. The procedure summarized in Exercise 40 will encompass the complete crossmatch procedure. Note that, when an "Immediate spin crossmatch" is required, the procedure will be terminated after that phase.

EXERCISE 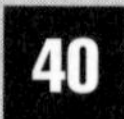 40 MAJOR CROSSMATCH

Using specimens provided by the instructor and labeled "donor" and "recipient," the student will perform the following procedure.

Equipment:
Gloves
Goggles
Recipient's sample
Donor's sample
10 × 75 or 12 × 75mm test tubes
Transfer pipets
0.85% saline in a wash bottle
LISS (or other enhancement media)
Anti-human globulin sera
Check cells
Marking pen
Serological centrifuge
Agglutination viewer
37°C heat block
Timer
Parafilm
Laboratory tissues
Beaker with disinfectant
Puncture-proof biohazard container

Procedure:

1. Wearing gloves and goggles, prepare a 5% cell suspension of recipient cells as outlined in Exercise 15.

EXERCISE 40 MAJOR CROSSMATCH *(continued)*

2. Perform ABO, Rh, and antibody screen with recipient's sample using procedures outlined in Exercises 17, 20, 22, and 30. It is not necessary to perform a weak D test on a recipient.

NOTE: The antibody screen may be performed with the compatibility test, depending on department protocol.

3. Choose a donor of the appropriate ABO and Rh type.

NOTE: If the recipient appears as Rh negative on immediate spin, choose Rh-negative blood for transfusion.

4. Using a segment from the donor unit, prepare a 5% suspension of donor's cells, as outlined in Exercise 15.
5. Label a tube with recipient identification.
6. Place 2 drops of recipient's serum into labeled tube.
7. Place 1 drop of donor cell suspension into the labeled tube.
8. Centrifuge for 15 seconds (or time designated for that centrifuge).
9. Read, interpret, and record results as "Immediate Spin." Remember to grade all reactions.

NOTE: If only the immediate spin phase is required, the unit may be labeled for transfusion. In addition, no hemolysis or agglutination indicates a "Compatible" unit at this phase of testing.

10. Add 2 drops of LISS (or other enhancement media) and incubate at 37°C for the time period established by the manufacturer. Set a timer.
11. Centrifuge, interpret, and record as "37° albumin."
12. Wash three or four times, as described in Exercise 13.
13. Add 2 drops of AHG sera. Centrifuge for 15 seconds (or the time designated for that centrifuge).
14. Using an agglutination viewer, read, interpret, and record results as "AHG."
15. Add 1 drop of check cells if the AHG phase was negative. Centrifuge.
16. Read, interpret, and record as "Check cells."
17. Overall interpretation of the crossmatch is **"Compatible"** if all phases are negative. If one or more phases shows hemolysis and/or agglutination, the crossmatch is "Incompatible" and the cause of the incompatibility must be investigated.
18. Discard all biohazardous waste into a puncture-proof biohazard container.

EMERGENCY CROSSMATCH PROCEDURE

Emergency situations in the blood bank may warrant the administration of red cells or whole blood in a short period of time. When this occurs, the units may either be transfused with no pretransfusion testing or with minimal testing. When units are distributed with no pretransfusion testing, O-negative units are most often transfused. The exception to this procedure is when the sex of the patient is known to be male and O-positive units may be given. O-positive units are more acceptable in male patients. If they develop anti-D after exposure to the antigen, it may create difficulty if emergency transfusions are required in the future, but hemolytic disease of the newborn is not a problem.

When time allows for typing of the recipient, a group and type of the patient is performed and group- and type-specific blood is released for transfusion. Complete compatibility testing is eventually done, no matter what the outcome of the situation.

CHOICE OF BLOOD TYPE FOR TRANSFUSION

Under ideal circumstances, each recipient receives ABO and Rh-specific transfusions. This is not always possible, and substitution may be necessary. Rh-positive individuals can always be transfused with Rh-negative cells. The reverse is not ideal. Rh-negative individuals may develop antibodies to the Rh antigen if transfused with Rh-positive blood. Women of childbearing age are protected from this immunization except under the most extreme emergency situations. In matters of life and death, Rh-positive cells may be transfused to Rh-negative individuals.

ABO substitution is done when necessary. The criteria for ABO group selection is made by determining if the cells will react with an antibody in the recipient's serum. If there is no possibility of reaction, then the cells are safe for transfusion. For example, a group AB individual has no anti-A in her serum and may be transfused with group A cells.

EXERCISE 41 EMERGENCY TRANSFUSION SITUATIONS

Students should work in pairs or small groups. Each pair or group should:

1. List at least five emergency situations that would require rapid treatment and may be encountered in the blood bank. Discuss each of these situations.
2. Have the instructor review the situations.
3. Interact with other pairs or groups and compile a list of situations.

CHOICE OF BLOOD WITH KNOWN ANTIBODY

After the appropriate ABO and Rh group has been chosen, atypical antibodies are considered. If one or more atypical antibodies is present, the units of cells for transfusion must be typed for the antigen that corresponds to the antibody in the serum. This is performed using the antigen typing procedures outlined in Unit 5.

RECORDS FOR COMPATIBILITY TESTING

In the blood bank, record keeping is imperative. Strict records of all test procedures and transfusions administered are maintained at all times. When performing compatibility tests, records of all test results are maintained. All test results are recorded and interpreted as the tests are completed.

Upon the completion of laboratory testing, units of blood being held for transfusion or transfused to a patient are labeled with the patient's identification and compatibility test results. Accurate recording of patient identification and test results is vital to preventing fatal transfusion errors. Labeling of the crossmatched units should be checked by a second person prior to transfusion to assure the accuracy of the patient identification. When releasing blood for transfusion, a system of multiple checks will help to prevent errors.

COMPONENTS

Units of blood for transfusion are drawn into containers that contain **anticoagulant/preservative** solutions. Anticoagulant/preservative solution varies depending on the manufacturer of the containers. The most common anticoagulant used is CPD (citrate phosphate dextrose) or its derivative. The purpose of the solution is to prevent the blood from clotting and to act as a preservative for the red cells. These two functions maintain the integrity of the cells in the units. Anticoagulant/preservative solutions are summarized in Table 7.1.

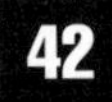

EXERCISE 42 LABELING UNITS FOR TRANSFUSION

Students will be provided with samples of labels used for units of blood to be transfused. Each student should:

1. Examine the label carefully and note all of the parts.
2. Diagram the label.
3. Complete the diagram with test results from a fictitious recipient.
4. Have the instructor check the work.

Table 7.1. Anticoagulant/Preservative Solutions for Blood Collection

Anticoagulant/Preservative	Shelf Life*
CPD	21 days
CPDA-1	35 days
Heparin	48 hours

*NOTE: Additives (AS-1 and AS-3) may extend the life of the red cells for up to 49 days from the day of collection.

Additive solution 1 (AS-1) and additive solution 3 (AS-3) may be used in combination with the anticoagulant/preservative solution. These additives extend the shelf life of the units of blood to as long as 49 days from collection, when used according to manufacturer's instructions.

COLLECTION OF WHOLE BLOOD UNITS

Collection of whole blood units is accomplished by qualified personnel using accepted phlebotomy procedures. The procedure must be performed using sterile equipment with a minimum of trauma to the integrity of the red cells.

TESTING OF DONOR UNITS

Each unit of whole blood is tested after collection. This testing is standard and includes the tests summarized in Table 7.2.

Donors found to have aberrant test results are notified and either deferred from donation or retested. Donors with positive results in hepatitis and HIV tests are deferred permanently. The blood from these donors must be discarded.

LABELING OF DONOR UNITS

Donor units are labeled as required by the Food and Drug Administration (FDA). Labeling takes place after all testing is completed and the unit is determined to be nonreactive for all of the tests performed. Units are then labeled with printed labels that contain the information summarized in Table 7.3.

Table 7.2. Tests Performed on Donor Blood

ABO group
Rh type
Weak D (if necessary)
Antibody screen
Hepatitis B surface antigen
Hepatitis C core antibody
Human immunodeficiency virus antibody I and II
Alanine aminotransferase (ALT)
Serologic test for syphilis (STS) (required only by the FDA)
HTLV I/II antibody
Hepatitis C virus antibody
Direct test for HIV antigen

Table 7.3. Information for Labeling Donor Blood

Name of the component
Kind and amount of anticoagulant
Volume of the unit
Required storage temperature
Name and address of collecting facility
Type of donor
Expiration date
Donor number
ABO group
Rh type
Antibody screen results
Additional test results are institution specific

COMPONENTS OF WHOLE BLOOD

Each unit of blood collected may be transfused as whole blood or split into components. These components may be transfused to different recipients as the need arises. Dividing a unit of whole blood into components is a common practice that optimizes the use of this resource. Components available for transfusion and some of their common uses are summarized in Table 7.4. Figure 7.2 summarizes some ways of dividing a unit to provided multiple components.

Table 7.4. Components Available for Transfusion

Component	Potential Recipients
Whole blood	Hemorrhage
Packed red cells*	Hemorrhage Anemia Surgical blood loss
Buffy-coat poor red cells	Anemia with sensitivity to white cells
Washed red cells	Anemia with sensitivity to white cells and/or plasma components
Frozen-thawed red cells†	Anemia with severe sensitivity to white cells and/or plasma components Transfusion to individuals with rare blood types or atypical antibodies Autologous storage
Fresh frozen plasma	Coagulation deficiencies Combined with massive red cell transfusion Disseminated intravascular coagulation
Stored plasma	Fluid replacement
Cryoprecipitate	Hemophiliacs Factor VIII and fibrinogen deficiency Disseminated intravascular coagulation
Platelet concentrate	Thrombocytopenia Consumption coagulopathy
Leukocyte concentrate	Severe leukopenia

*Also known as packed cells (PC), concentrated red cells (CRC), packed red blood cells (PRBC).
†Also known as frozen deglycerolized red cells.

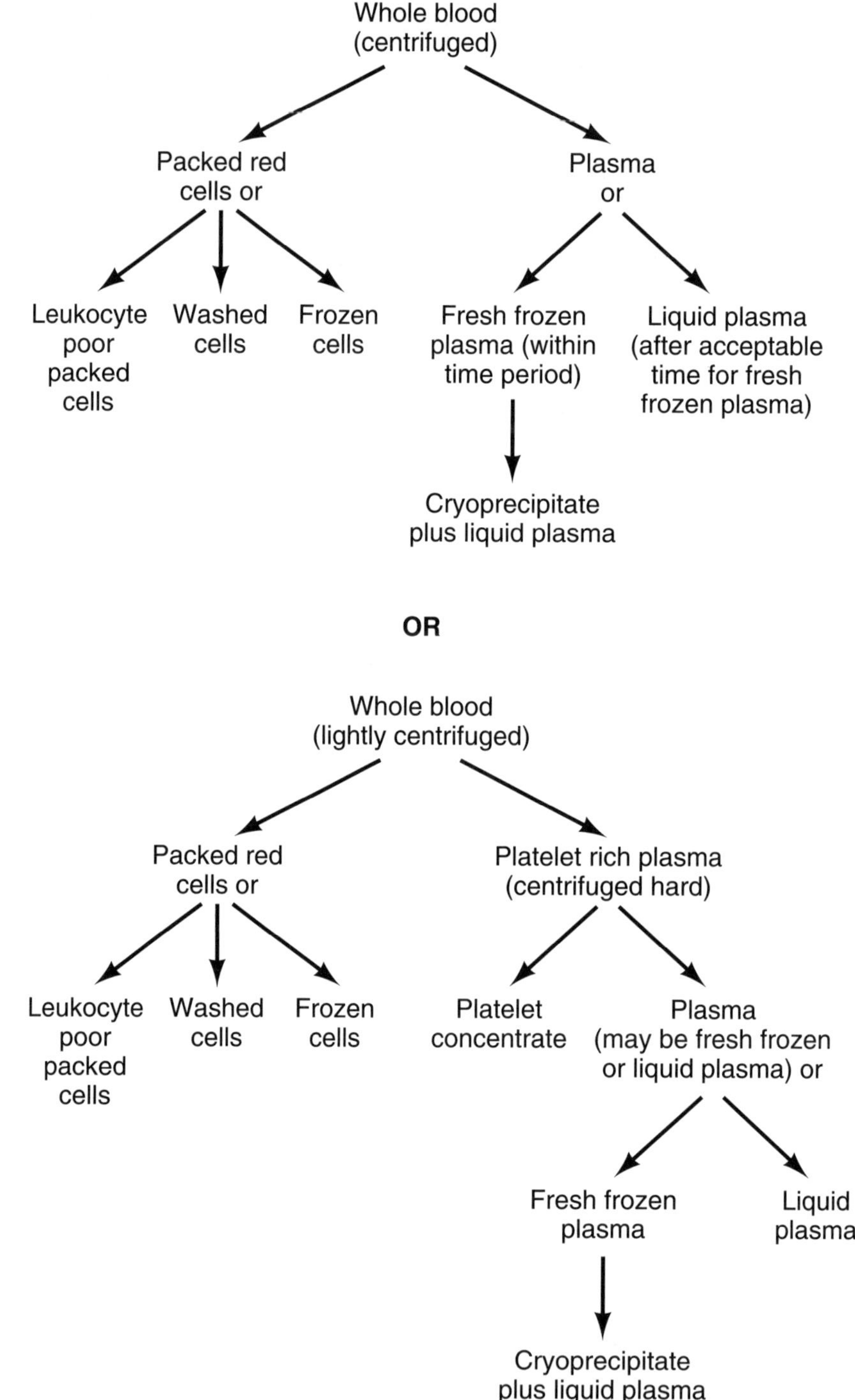

fig. 7.2. Component preparation from a single unit of whole blood.

COMPONENT PREPARATION

Component preparation is usually performed in the donor center, but a technician may need to prepare or pool some products for transfusion. Methods of preparation vary by institution, and the operating procedures for that institution should be consulted. It should be noted that vital steps in component preparation include maintaining sterility and labeling the container after the preparation is complete.

Packed Red Blood Cells

Preparation of all components begins with a unit of whole blood. The primary component prepared from a unit of whole blood is packed red cells. In order to prepare packed cells, the units of whole blood must be allowed to settle by gravity or be centrifuged. The unit is processed and the plasma removed. These red cells may be processed and transfused as packed red cells or may be converted to washed or frozen red cells.

Leukocyte Poor Red Cells

Leukocyte poor red cells may be produced by several methods. Washed and **frozen thawed** or **deglycerolized red cells** are two methods to remove large numbers of the white blood cells. Additionally, units of packed cells may be filtered or packed using an inverted centrifugation method. See Figure 7.3 for a description of inverted centrifugation.

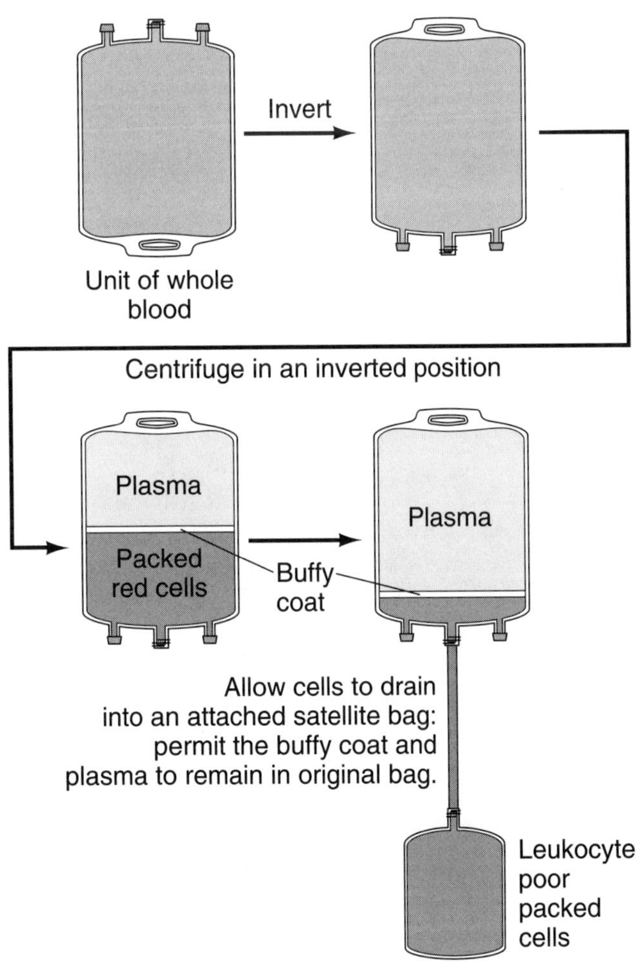

fig. 7.3. Preparation of leukocyte poor red cells from a unit of whole blood using inverted centrifugation.

Cryoprecipitate

Cryoprecipitate is a product prepared from plasma that is removed from red cells soon after collection. It is a concentrate of coagulation factors VIII and I (fibrinogen). The product is prepared by removing the plasma from red cells and freezing to a slushy mixture. At that point, a "button" of concentrated material in the bottom of the plasma is the cryoprecipitate. The remaining plasma is removed and the button of cryprecipitate labeled and frozen.

Plasma

Fresh frozen plasma (FFP) is the most common form of transfused plasma issued by the blood bank. It is labeled "fresh frozen plasma" because it is removed from whole blood and frozen within 6 hours of collection. It provides a source of coagulation factors.

Single donor plasma or **liquid plasma** is the second source of plasma for transfusion. This plasma is used for fluid replacement since it is either not collected within the time frame for fresh frozen plasma or has had the cryoprecipitate removed.

Platelet Concentrate

Platelet concentrate may be prepared by lightly spinning the whole blood to allow the platelets to remain in the plasma. The plasma is removed and centrifuged. At this point, the platelets are located in the bottom of the bag. The remaining plasma is removed and may be frozen. If this is done within the 6-hour time frame the plasma will be fresh frozen plasma. Otherwise, the plasma is stored plasma. For a summary of this procedure see Figure 7.4.

Multiple units of platelet concentrate may be collected from a single donor by pheresis. This provides the patient with platelets from one donor. This reduces the exposure to foreign antibodies and the possibility of developing unexpected antibodies.

Leukocyte Concentrate

Leukocyte concentrate is collected by **pheresis**. This component is then stored and transfused as needed by patients. For additional information on pheresis, the inquisitive student is referred to a textbook on Immunohematology.

STORAGE OF COMPONENTS

Each component has an expiration date and maximum storage time. Acceptable storage times and temperatures are established by licensing and accrediting agencies. These storage times and temperatures are summarized in Table 7.5.

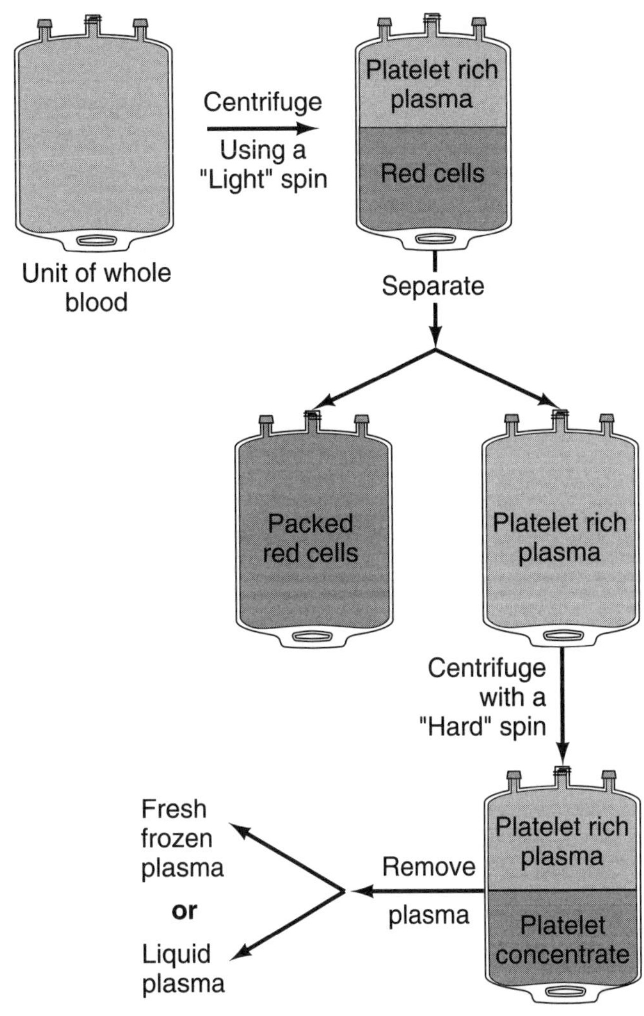

fig. 7.4. Preparation of platelet concentration from a unit of whole blood using centrifugation.

EXERCISE 43 COMPONENT PREPARATION

A student representative or instructor should contact a local donor center and arrange for a visit. If this is not possible, the students should do the following alternate assignment:

1. Choose a component discussed in the previous sections.
2. Research that component with references provided by the instructor.
3. Prepare a poster outlining the component and its preparation method.
4. Share the poster with the class.
5. Display the posters in a prominent place.

Table 7.5. Storage Times and Temperatures for Components

Component	Storage Time	Storage Temperature
Whole blood	21 to 42 days (anticoagulant/additive dependent‡)	1°C–6°C
Red cells*	21 to 42 days (closed system) (anticoagulant/additive dependent‡)	1°C–6°C
Washed red cells	24 hours after washing	1°C–6°C
Frozen red cells	10 years†	<−65°C
Thawed deglycerolized cells	24 hours after thawing	1°C–6°C
Fresh frozen plasma	12 months	<−18°C
Single donor or liquid plasma	Up to 5 days after expiration of original unit or 12 months	1°C–6°C or <−18°C
Thawed fresh frozen plasma	24 hours	1°C–6°C
Cryoprecipitate	12 months	<−18°C
Thawed cryoprecipitate	6 hours	20°C–24°C
Platelet concentrate	72 or 120 hours (container dependent)	20°C–24°C
Leukocyte concentrate	Up to 24 hours	20°C–24°C

*Using an open system, the cells outdate 24 hours after preparation.
†Rare blood has been stored longer and used with reduced red cell harvest.
‡Anticoagulant specific storage times: ACD and CPD—21 days; CPDA-1—35 days; AS-1 and AS-3—42 days.

SUMMARY

Compatibility testing prior to transfusion is an important aspect of day-to-day operations in the blood bank. Technicians are responsible for performing test procedures and preparing the units for distribution to the recipients. Immediate spin or complete crossmatches are performed prior to transfusion for each recipient. The clerical aspects of compatibility testing are vital to avoid transfusion reactions.

Choice of correct group and type are essential for successful tranfusion. The technician must be familiar with emergency transfusion procedures and guidelines for switching types when employed in the blood bank.

Additionally, the components available for transfusion are diverse and originate from whole blood. Each unit may be divided into components that may be used by multiple recipients rather than transfusing a single unit of whole blood to a single patient. These components include packed red cells, leukocyte-poor cell products, platelet concentrate, leukocyte concentrate, cryoprecipitate, and plasma.

Collection, preparation, and storage of these components is the responsibility of donor and distribution centers and helps to provide optimal healthcare to the individuals requiring transfusion. Distribution of components for transfusion falls into the responsibility of the technician working in the blood bank.

CASE STUDY 7

A trauma center received several casualties from a multicar automobile accident. One casualty was an 18-year-old female with internal injuries. In preparation for surgery, the surgeon requested 10 units of blood to be crossmatched for transfusion. The surgeon wanted 2 units to be started immediately. The technician collected a sample, but time was insufficient to perform an ABO and Rh type before releasing the first 2 units. Respond to the following questions related to this case.

QUESTIONS

1. What ABO and Rh type should be chosen for the 2 units to be transfused immediately?
2. As soon as the sample has clotted and can be used for testing, what tests will be performed on this sample?
3. After the 2 emergency units have been released, will any tests need to be performed with these units? If so, what are they?

CASE STUDY 8

A leukemia patient is admitted to the local hospital. The patient was experiencing fatigue and a localized infection that had not been receptive to antibiotics. The hematologist ordered a complete blood count and coagulation testing. The results reflected decreased values for the red blood cell count, white blood cell count, and platelet count. The coagulation tests reflected normal levels of coagulation factors. This patient had been previously transfused. When the records were checked, fever and chills were noted with previous red cell transfusions. The director of the blood bank had reviewed these records and indicated that the cause was probably a sensitivity to white blood cells.

QUESTIONS

1. Does this patient need transfusion therapy? If so, what components?
2. What consideration needs to be given to the sensitivity to white blood cells? Does this information alter the type of red cell component chosen?
3. What component may help to fight the unresponsive infection?
4. Is the decreased platelet count significant for transfusion therapy? Why or why not?

CASE STUDY 9

A donor center has recruited donors for a bloodmobile visit at a local church. Fifty donors have arrived as the blood drive begins. A technician begins to process a donor who tells the technician that previous tests showed a positive test for hepatitis B. The donor has B-negative blood, and that is a type that is in demand. The donor insists that her blood was accepted for transfusion on her last visit and that she wants to donate. The technician collects the unit of blood and labels it with a donor number. There were extra donor labels. The technician neglected to discard the extra labels but rather left them at the drawing station.

QUESTIONS

1. What information should this technician give to the donor?
2. Will the blood from this donor be used for transfusion? Why or why not?
3. Did the technician make an error when labeling the unit? If so, what was it?

REVIEW QUESTIONS

1. Major crossmatch consists of
   a. donor's serum and recipient's cells
   b. donor's serum and donor's cells
   c. recipient's serum and donor's cells
   d. recipient's serum and recipient's cells
2. Immediate spin crossmatch detects incompatibility with
   a. ABO group
   b. Rh types
   c. AHG reactive antibodies
   d. hemolytic antibodies
3. Leukocyte poor red blood cells are prepared by all methods below except
   a. filtering
   b. freezing
   c. packing
   d. washing
4. FFP may be stored
   a. 1 year at 1°C to 6°C
   b. 1 year at $<^{-}18$°C
   c. 5 years at 1°C to 6°C
   d. 5 years at $<^{-}18$°C

5. Deglycerolized red blood cells may be transfused to individuals who require a red blood cell transfusion but also
   a. have coagulation deficiencies
   b. are allergic to anticoagulant
   c. are sensitized to white blood cells
   d. need platelet concentrate
6. An additive to extend the life of whole blood is
   a. AS-3
   b. CPD
   c. CPD-A1
   d. heparin
7. Packed red blood cells prepared in an open system will expire in
   a. 24 hours
   b. 72 hours
   c. 21 days
   d. 35 days
8. When labeling donor units, the information that is *not* required on the label is
   a. anticoagulant/preservative solution used
   b. date of collection
   c. name of collection facility
   d. volume of blood collected
9. Cryoprecipitate contains
   a. platelets
   b. white blood cells
   c. leukocyte poor red blood cells
   d. coagulation factors VIII and I
10. When performing a compatibility test, agglutination is noted in the AHG phase. This test should be interpreted as
   a. compatible
   b. incompatible
   c. inconclusive

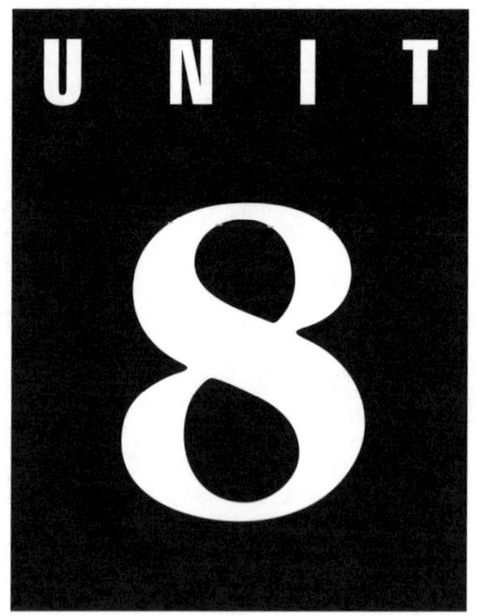

Hemolytic Disease of the Newborn, Transfusion Reactions, and Autoimmune Hemolytic Anemia

LEARNING OBJECTIVES

After studying this unit, it is the responsibility of the student to know the following objectives:

- **Define terms listed in the glossary.**
- **Outline criteria for diagnosis and treatment of hemolytic disease of the newborn.**
- **Perform tests to diagnose presence of hemolytic disease of the newborn.**
- **Describe common categories of transfusion reactions.**
- **Perform a transfusion reaction investigation.**
- **Discuss prevention of hemolytic transfusion reaction.**
- **Outline causes of autoimmune hemolytic anemia.**
- **Briefly discuss transfusion therapy in patients with autoimmune hemolytic anemia.**

GLOSSARY

amniocentesis procedure for removing amniotic fluid for analysis.

anaphylactic intense allergic reaction, including bronchial constriction and collapse.

anemia decreased oxygen-carrying capacity due to low hemoglobin level.

antenatal before birth.

autoimmune hemolytic anemia (AIHA) clinical condition of immune origin with hemolysis of red cells and a resulting anemia.

exchange transfusion transfusion of cells performed after birth that uses a system where some of the infant's cells are removed for each portion of transfused cells that are administered.

febrile having a fever.

fetomaternal hemorrhage fetal bleeding into the maternal circulation.

hemoglobinemia presence of free hemoglobin in the serum or plasma.

hemolysis destruction of red blood cells with release of hemoglobin.

hemolytic disease of the newborn (HDN) clinical condition involving the fetus and the neonate that results in hemolysis of red cells due to maternal antibody coating the red cells of the baby.

hemolytic transfusion reaction (HTR) adverse reaction to transfusion, most often resulting from an interaction between antigens of the donor and antibodies of the recipient.

hypothermia decrease in body temperature.

in utero while the fetus is in the uterus.

intrauterine transfusion transfusion administered to a fetus still in the uterus.

Kleihauer-Betke acid elution stain stain with a low pH that will stain fetal cells a dark pink while causing the adult cells to lyse and appear as pale-staining ghost cells.

parallel testing tests performed in the same manner with multiple samples.

phototherapy treatment using lights.

postpartum after giving birth.

posttransfusion after transfusion.

pretransfusion before transfusion.

qualitative establishes presence of a substance but does not determine the quantity.

quantitative determines the amount of substance present.

Rh immune globulin concentrated anti-D commercially processed for administration to prevent Rh hemolytic disease of the newborn.

rosette clump of cells consisting of a central cell surrounded by other cells.

sepsis presence of bacterial infection in the circulatory system.

titer amount of an antibody in a fluid; determined by performing a series of dilutions on the fluid.

transfusion reaction untoward effect of transfusion.

urticaria hives.

Wharton's jelly sticky connective tissue substance found on the umbilical cord.

INTRODUCTION

Test methods discussed in the previous units are helpful in diagnosing and monitoring treatment of certain clinical conditions. Conditions that present with positive antibody screens and direct antiglobulin tests include **hemolytic disease of the newborn (HDN)**, **hemolytic transfusion reactions (HTR),** and **autoimmune hemolytic anemia (AIHA).** These conditions will be briefly discussed and methods for performing diagnostic tests outlined.

HEMOLYTIC DISEASE OF THE NEWBORN

Hemolytic disease of the newborn (HDN) is a condition that involves hemolysis of red cells in the fetus and neonate. In order for HDN to occur, an antibody must be present in the mother that corresponds to an antigen on the surface of the red cells of the fetus. While ***in utero,*** the antibody crosses the placenta, attaches to the antigens, and hemolyzes the red cells of the fetus. This provides a situation of danger for the baby both *in utero* and after birth. HDN may be placed into three categories. These are summarized in Table 8.1.

ABO hemolyic disease of the newborn is the most commonly seen, but Rh hemolytic disease is usually the most severe. Hemolytic disease of the newborn caused by other antibodies is uncommon, but may be severe. Antibodies, other than ABO antibodies and anti-Rh_o(D), that may cause HDN are summarized in Table 8.2.

ABO HEMOLYTIC DISEASE OF THE NEWBORN

Hemolytic disease of the newborn (HDN) caused by ABO antibodies is the most common type of HDN. The antibodies are those that are found in the maternal circulation. The antibodies cross the placenta and attach to the red cells of the infant if the corresponding antigen is present. The most common scenario for ABO hemolytic disease is a group O mother and a group A infant, although other combinations are possible. The testing and investigation is the same as for Rh hemolytic disease.

Table 8.1. Categories of Hemolytic Disease of the Newborn

Rh HDN (Anti-Rh_o[D])
ABO HDN
HDN caused by other antibodies

Table 8.2. Antibodies Other than ABO Which May Cause Hemolytic Disease of the Newborn

Rh antibodies	Kell system antibodies	Duffy system antibodies	Kidd system antibodies	MNSs system antibodies
Anti-C	Anti-K	Anti-Fy^a	Anti-Jk^a	Anti-S
Anti-E	Anti-k	Anti-Fy^b	Anti-Jk^b	Anti-s
Anti-c				
Anti-e				

ABO hemolytic disease is often less severe than Rh, but may require treatment. **Phototherapy** or an **exchange transfusion** is sometimes necessary.

Rh HEMOLYTIC DISEASE OF THE NEWBORN

A typical scenario for Rh HDN is summarized in Table 8.3. Rh HDN is diagnosed by testing all expectant mothers. ABO, Rh, and an antibody screen will be performed. If anti-D is found in the serum, the physician will perform antibody screen and **titer** tests on the mother throughout the pregnancy.

Antibody Titers

Antibody titer is determined by performing a set of serial dilutions using the mother's serum and reacting the diluted serum with Rh-positive cells. Each time a titer is performed, a serum sample is used. For the sake of comparison, a second titer is performed using a frozen portion of serum from the previous titer. This is known as **parallel testing**. For an example of a titer with results, see Figure 8.1.

Table 8.3. Findings in Rh Hemolytic Disease of the Newborn

Mother	Baby
D and weak D negative	D or weak D positive
Antibody screen positive for anti-D	Direct antiglobulin test positive
	Anti-D found in eluate

EXERCISE 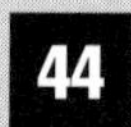 44 DETERMINATION OF Rh ANTIBODIES IN EXPECTANT MOTHERS

Using a sample provided by the instructor, each student will perform the following tests and answer the questions. Be certain to follow all safety precautions for handling biohazards.

Tests:
ABO (Exercises 17 and 20)
Rh and weak D, if indicated (Exercises 22 and 23)
Antibody Screen (Exercise 30)
Antibody identification panel, if indicated (Exercise 32)

1. Does this mother have the criteria to produce a baby that may have Rh HDN? Explain.
2. If the answer to question #1 is yes, what criteria must be present in the infant in order for this to happen?
3. What type of eluate may be effective for extracting the Rh antibody from the cells of the baby?

	Dilution Strength							
	1:1	1:2	1:4	1:8	1:16	1:32	1:64	1:128
Sample #1	4+	4+	3+	2+	1+	0	0	0
Sample #2 (4 weeks later)	4+	4+	4+	3+	2+	1+	1+	0

fig. 8.1. Sample titer results from a serum containing Anti-Rh_o(D).

As the pregnancy progresses and titers are performed, the physician is looking for an increase in the level of the titer. A significant change is when the titer increases by two tubes or more. If the titer remains stable, the fetus most likely does not have the antigen that corresponds to the antibody in the maternal serum.

If the titer significantly increases, decisions on treatment of the baby must be made. Interventions such as **intrauterine transfusion** may be used before birth, whereas exchange transfusion is a treatment option after birth. For either of these procedures, crossmatch is performed using the mother's serum since that is the origin of the antibody.

TESTING OF NEONATES

Newborn infants are tested using either the cord blood or a capillary sample collected from the heel. The testing of cord blood samples is common and resembles normal cell testing with one exception. **Wharton's jelly,** a connective tissue substance in the umbilical cord, may contaminate the samples. When this contamination occurs, the sticky nature of the Wharton's jelly may cause false-positive agglutination. In order to prevent this, the cells from the cord blood sample must be very thoroughly washed with isotonic saline prior to use for testing.

The cord blood or capillary sample is tested for ABO forward grouping, Rh typing, and direct antiglobulin testing. If the DAT is positive, an eluate may be performed on the sample. Remember that reverse grouping is not performed on neonates, since the infant has not developed antibodies.

EXERCISE 45 TITER INTERPRETATIONS

The instructor will provide each group of students with results from one or more titers. The group will do the following:

1. Evaluate the test results.
2. Determine if there is a change in titer and whether or not it is significant.
3. Discuss possible treatment options for the infant.

EXERCISE 46 TESTING OF CORD BLOOD SAMPLES

Each student will be provided with a cord blood or simulated sample provided by the instructor. Each student should wash the sample a minimum of six times, using the procedure in Exercise 15. Then the student should perform the tests listed in the previous section and interpret the results. The student should be certain to use all safety precautions for protection from biohazards.

PREVENTION OF Rh HEMOLYTIC DISEASE OF THE NEWBORN

It is possible to prevent most cases of Rh HDN by careful monitoring of Rh-negative pregenant women. The development of **Rh immune globulin** aided in reducing the number of cases of Rh HDN by preventing development of anti-D in the mother. Criteria for administration of Rh immune globulin are summarized in Table 8.4.

Rh Immmune Globulin

Rh immune globulin (RhIg) is concentrated anti-D. This antibody is a human product commercially purified, titered, and packaged for sale under trade names. The product is administered to Rh-negative women who have antibody screens negative for anti-D. The presence of other antibodies does not preclude the adminstration of this product.

The mechanism of RhIg is coating of the Rh-positive fetal cells in the maternal circulation by the anti-D. The antibody-coated cells are recognized by the mother's system as abnormal and removed from the circulation. This prevents the maternal immune system from having the opportunity to process the antigens on the surface of the fetal cells. Hence, no antibody is formed.

Rh immune globulin is packaged in 300 μg doses for use with any pregnancy progressing beyond the first trimester. A 300-μg dose will counteract up to 30 ml of Rh-positive whole blood. The dose is routinely administered twice: at 28 weeks' gestation **(antenatal)** and within 72 hours after the birth of an Rh-positive infant **(postpartum).**

Rh immune globulin is also administered following the termination of any pregnancy and after **amniocentesis** in an Rh-negative mother. Small doses are packaged to be administered up to the end of the first trimester.

Table 8.4. Criteria for Administration of Rh Immune Globulin

Mother	Infant
Rh negative, weak D negative Antibody screen negative for anti-D	Rh positive (or potentially Rh positive)

EXERCISE 47 Rh IMMUNE GLOBULIN

In small groups, the students will read the package insert from a package of Rh immune globulin. Each group will answer the following questions.

1. What is the source of this product?
2. What is the volume of fluid in each vial?
3. How is the solution administered?
4. What are the potential side effects of the product?
5. Are there any contraindications for receiving this product?
6. In what situation(s) other than the pregnancy of an Rh-negative mother may Rh immune globulin be used?

DETERMINING DOSAGE OF Rh IMMUNE GLOBULIN

Events may occur either before or during delivery that may result in more than 30 ml of fetal blood passing into the maternal circulation **(fetomaternal hemorrhage).** When this happens, greater than one vial of Rh immune globulin is required to prevent the mother from developing the anti-D antibody. Tests are available to determine whether an excessive bleed has occurred. These tests include: fetal screen and **Kleihauer-Betke acid elution stain** (both available in kit form). The fetal screen is a **qualitative** test, whereas the acid elution stain may be quantitated.

Fetal Screen Methods

Fetal screen kits use a method that produces **rosettes** in a positive test. A maternal sample of either clotted or anticoagulated blood is used. The cells are incubated with anti-D. This allows attachment of the antibody to any fetal cells in the sample. Following incubation, the cells are washed to remove excess antibody. Indicator cells are added to the washed patient sample. The indicator cells are Rh-positive cells. If fetal cells have attached to antibody during the incubation, the Rh-positive indicator cells will attach to the free arm of the anti-D molecules that are attached to the fetal cells. This binding of the indicator cells will occur so that they surround the fetal cells and appear as a rosette. See Figure 8.2 for a pictorial explanation of rosette formation.

After the addition of indicator cells, the mixture is centrifuged and examined microscopically. The appearance of rosettes is considered a positive result. Positive and negative controls are used. When interpreting the patient's test results, a comparison to the controls is made. A **quantitative** test method is performed on all positive fetal screens.

Kleihauer-Betke Acid Elution Stain

The Kleihauer-Betke acid elution stain is a quantitative method for determining the amount of fetomaternal hemorrhage. The method consists of a buffer with an acid pH. When applied to thin smears of a maternal sample, this buffer will cause

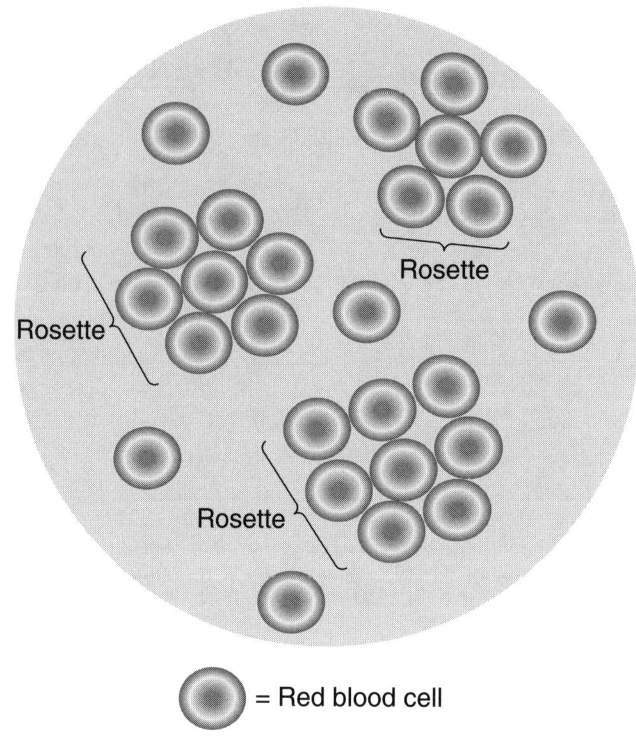

fig. 8.2. Rosette formation in a fetal screen test.

EXERCISE 48 FETAL SCREEN TEST

Each student (or small group of students) should be provided with a fetal screen test kit and a patient sample. The test should be performed following the instructions from the package insert. Results are recorded and the following questions considered. Be certain to follow all safety precautions for prevention of exposure to biohazards.

1. Did the patient have a fetomaternal hemorrhage?
2. Is further testing necessary? If so, describe the tests.
3. What implications does this have for future pregnancies for this patient?

the adult cells to lose their hemoglobin. The hemoglobin in fetal cells will be resistant to this loss of hemoglobin. The smear is then stained. Adult cells will appear as pale ghost cells, whereas the fetal cells will stain dark pink. The percentage of fetal cells is determined and used to calculate the number of vials of Rh immune globulin necessary. See Figure 8.3 for a visual comparison of fetal and adult cells in an acid elution procedure.

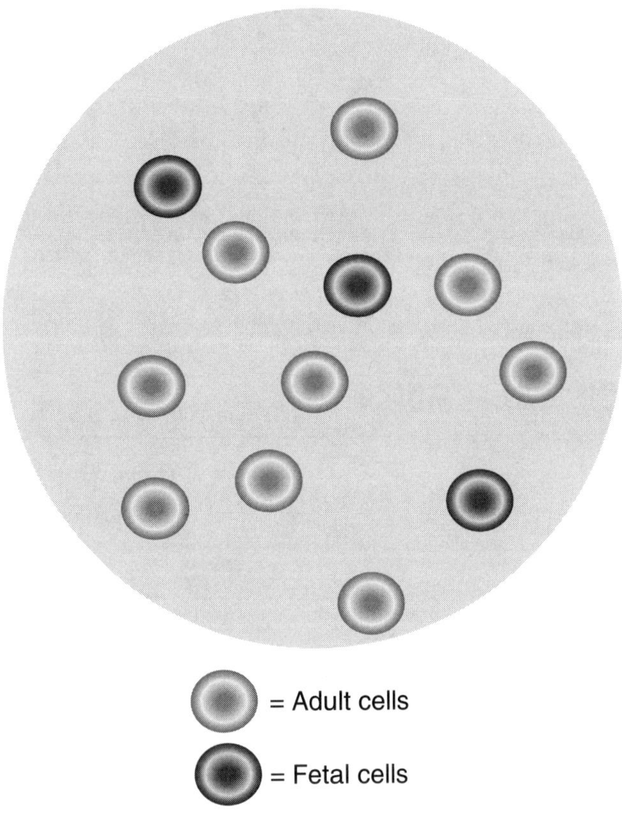

fig. 8.3. Kleihauer-Betke staining of fetal and adult cells. Fetal cells stain dark while the adult cells are pale ghost cells.

EXERCISE 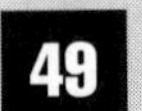

QUANTITATION OF FETAL-MATERNAL HEMORRHAGE

Each student is provided with smears from an acid elution stain test. The student should examine the smears using oil immersion.

1. Count 2000 cells and differentiate the number of fetal cells in the total.

NOTE: Count all cells in a field with a hand tally counter. Count the fetal cells a second time as a separate count and record separately. Repeat for each field.

2. Determine the percentage of cells that are fetal cells.
3. Calculate the total volume of fetal maternal hemorrhage by multiplying the percentage of fetal cells by 50.
4. Determine the number of vials of Rh immune globulin necessary for this patient. Remember that each vial counteracts 30 ml of fetal blood.

HEMOLYTIC DISEASE OF THE NEWBORN CAUSED BY OTHER ANTIBODIES

Any blood group system in which the antigen is well developed in the fetus and neonate and antibodies of the IgG class are produced may be implicated in hemolytic disease of the newborn. These antigen systems are summarized in Table 8.2. Diagnosis of these cases of HDN is identical to that previously discussed. It should be noted, however, that Rh immune globulin will not prevent HDN caused by these antibodies.

TRANSFUSION REACTIONS

A **transfusion reaction** is defined as any untoward effect of a transfusion of blood or blood product. Results of transfusion reactions range from slight symptoms to death. Major categories of transfusion reactions are summarized in Table 8.5.

HEMOLYTIC TRANSFUSION REACTIONS

The most severe and dreaded transfusion reaction results from acute hemolysis of donor's red cells as they enter the circulation of the recipient. This is known as an immediate or acute hemolytic transfusion reaction. It is usually caused by an ABO incompatibility, which most frequently results from some form of clerical error. The investigation of transfusion reaction centers around the hemolytic transfusion reaction. The causes of many other types of transfusion reactions cannot be investigated by serological testing.

A delayed hemolytic transfusion reaction is a hemolytic reaction that may occur up to 14 days after the transfusion. Delayed reactions most often result from an anamnestic antibody response. The symptoms are often mild and may go unnoticed, but death has occurred from delayed transfusion reactions.

Table 8.5. Categories of Transfusion Reactions

Categories of Transfusion Reactions
Hemolytic
Immediate
Delayed
Allergic
Anaphylactic
Urticarial
Infectious disease
Hepatitis
HIV
Protozoal infection
Sexually transmitted diseases
Cytomegalovirus
Circulatory overload
Alloimmunization
Graft vs. host disease
Iron overload
Febrile reactions
Reaction to bacterial contamination

OTHER CATEGORIES OF TRANSFUSION REACTIONS

One of the most common forms of transfusion reaction is the **febrile** reaction. This reaction exhibits the symptoms of fever and chills and is frequently caused by antibodies to antigens on white cells or platelets. While uncomfortable for the patient, this type of transfusion reaction is not life-threatening but does require terminating the transfusion. Future transfusions may require leukocyte-poor packed red cells.

Allergic reactions vary from very mild cases of **urticaria** or hives to life-threatening **anaphylactic** reactions. Urticarial reactions may be caused by multiple factors, and the causes are usually not determined. Treatment with antihistamines and continuing the transfusion are appropriate. An anaphylactic reaction happens very rapidly as the transfusion begins. It requires immediate intervention. The cause is usually a rapid antibody reaction to a plasma protein lacking in the recipient. Future transfusions require the use of cells with no plasma. Frozen-thawed cells are the best choice.

Infrequent causes of reactions include gram-negative **sepsis** caused by contaminated units, **hypothermia** caused by rapid transfusion of cold blood, and circulatory overload induced by rapid transfusion of blood into individuals unable to tolerate the fluid. These infrequent reactions are not detectable serologically and cannot be detected in the laboratory investigation of transfusion reactions.

INVESTIGATION OF TRANSFUSION REACTIONS

Investigation of transfusion reactions centers around detecting a hemolytic reaction. The process of investigation varies by institution. A general system for investigation is discussed in the text and summarized in a flowchart in Figure 8.4

RESPONSE TO TRANSFUSION REACTION

Technicians will not usually be involved in detecting the symptoms of a transfusion reaction nor will they take the immediate steps to stop the transfusion and begin investigation or treatment. As soon as a transfusion reaction is suspected, the transfusion is stopped and a physician notified. The intravenous line is kept open and saline is infused. The blood bank will be notified at this point. Either the appropriate specimens will be collected and sent to the laboratory or laboratory personnel will collect the samples.

IDENTIFICATION CHECK

The identification of the patient and unit for transfusion are checked at the bedside. If a discrepancy is determined, this is documented and reported to the physician. Clerical identification is checked again in the laboratory and all information documented.

SAMPLE COLLECTION

Samples collected vary by institution. Commonly, a plain nonanticoagulated tube and an EDTA tube are collected. Care is taken to prevent **hemolysis** dur-

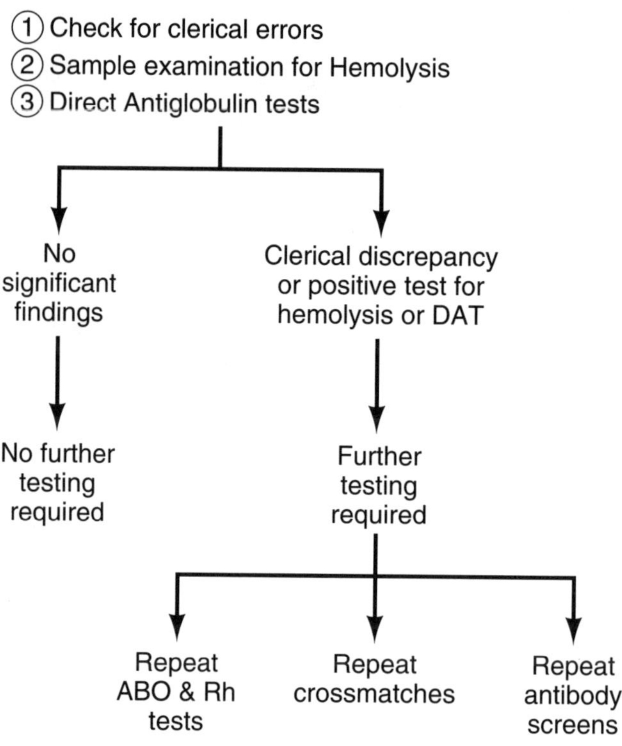

fig. 8.4. Laboratory investigation of transfusion reactions.

ing collection. The unit of blood with all infusion sets and tubing attached is also forwarded to the blood bank with all of the proper labels and forms. Urine samples and a bacterial culture of the blood bag may also be required.

TEST PROCEDURES

Visual examination of all samples for hemolysis occurs after centrifugation. Red and pink plasma or serum indicates **hemoglobinemia.** If hemoglobinemia is present in the **posttransfusion** sample but not in the **pretransfusion** sample, an intense investigation ensues.

Direct antiglobulin testing is also part of the immediate investigation of transfusion reaction. A DAT is performed on the posttransfusion sample. This test may be positive with a mixed field reaction if an immune reaction is occurring in the patient. If the reacting cells are being rapidly cleared from the system, the DAT may be negative.

FURTHER TESTING

If evidence exists of a clerical error such as misidentification, hemolysis exists in the posttransfusion sample, or the posttransfusion DAT is positive, an intense investigation is necessary. The testing performed in this investigation is summarized in Table 8.6. If all of these items are negative with no controversy encountered, the investigation is stopped since no immune cause seems to be present. If all initial tests are negative and the physician still detects symptoms of a hemolytic transfusion reaction, the remaining steps of the testing process may be necessary.

Table 8.6. Tests for Investigation of Transfusion Reaction

ABO and Rh Tests	Compatibility Testing	Antibody Screen
Patient's pretransfusion sample	Pretransfusion sample and donor segment	Pretransfusion sample
Patient's posttransfusion sample	Posttransfusion sample and donor segment	Posttransfusion sample
Donor segment		Donor segment

EXERCISE 

INVESTIGATION OF A TRANSFUSION REACTION

In small groups, students will perform a transfusion reaction investigation. The group should perform the following determinations and then answer the questions that follow. Be certain to follow all precautions of prevention of exposure to biohazards.

1. Compare labels on pretransfusion sample, posttransfusion sample, and transfused unit. Record all observations.
2. Observe the centrifuged samples for hemoglobinemia. Record all observations.
3. Perform direct antiglobulin tests on pretransfusion and posttransfusion samples.
4. Decide if it is possible that a hemolytic transfusion reaction has occurred. If the potential for hemolysis exists, continue with the exercises that follow, otherwise answer the questions.
5. Perform ABO and Rh on the pretransfusion sample, posttransfusion sample, and donor unit. Record all observations.
6. Decide if discrepancies exist. Record all observations.
7. Repeat the major compatibility test using the pretransfusion sample and the posttransfusion sample. Record all observations.
8. Decide if discrepancies exist. Record all observations.

QUESTIONS

1. Did you continue after step #4? Why or why not? Did you make the correct decision?
2. Were discrepancies encountered in any of the steps after #4? If so, what were they?
3. Did any clerical errors occur? If so, did they cause the reaction?
4. If the reaction was not hemolytic, was it possible to determine the cause? Why or why not?

AUTOIMMUNE HEMOLYTIC ANEMIA

Autoimmune hemolytic anemia (AIHA) is a clinical condition that is a primary condition or secondary to a separate condition. In AIHA, the immune system malfunctions and allows the body to produce an autoantibody against antigens on the patient's red cells. This causes hemolysis and **anemia.** The mechanism goes against Landsteiner's law, since the antibody is directed against an antigen that *is* present on the red cells.

TEST RESULTS IN AIHA

The most remarkable test in autoimmune hemolytic anemia is the positive direct antiglobulin test. This test may be positive with any antiglobulin sera, depending on the substance coating the red cells. The coating substance may be immunoglobulin, complement, or both. The antibody screen cells may be positive due to excess autoantibody that has "spilled over" into the serum or a separate alloantibody. The antibody may be identifiable with an antibody identification panel or may be nonspecific so that no pattern is seen. Be aware that when these cells are tested with AHG, a positive result will occur. This includes the autocontrol in the antibody screen and antibody identification, as well as antigen-typing tests that use AHG. Whenever the autocontrol appears positive, the technician should perform a DAT test to confirm that a substance is coating the cells. The use of more than one type of AHG sera will help to determine the specificity of the coating substance.

DRUG-INDUCED AIHA

Medications may cause AIHA. There are four mechanisms that cause drug-induced AIHA. The antibody is usually nonspecific and antibody identification will provide no pattern of reactivity. Drug-induced AIHA can be diagnosed with a thorough medical history. Removal of the medication will usually correct the situation.

TRANSFUSION OF PATIENTS WITH AIHA

The technician may need to provide transfusions for patients with AIHA. Frequently, the crossmatches will be incompatible and a physician will determine whether transfusion is necessary. ABO and Rh-specific blood will be transfused, even if incompatible.

It is best not to transfuse unless the situation is life-threatening. The transfusion of cells will sometimes provide more cells to hemolyze and compound the problem.

SUMMARY

Hemolytic disease of the newborn, transfusion reaction, and autoimmune hemolytic anemia are the three conditions discussed in this unit. These clinical conditions impact on the workload of the technician. Hemolytic disease of the newborn requires testing and treatment of both the mother and the neonate. Blood bank technicians perform tests and provide information to physicians to make diagnoses and future treatment decisions.

Transfusion reactions are the sole responsibility of the blood bank, since the transfusion originated in that department. The technician must recognize the serological signs of hemolytic transfusion reaction. Follow-up of all untoward reactions is important for best patient care. The follow-up procedures include clerical checks and serological and bacterial tests. These procedures are useful in the diagnosis of a hemolytic transfusion reaction but are not very effective in the diagnosis of other types of reactions.

Autoimmune hemolytic anemia may be a primary or secondary condition. It is a condition in which the body is producing antibodies directed at the antigens on the surface of the red cells. Diagnosis requires the use of the direct antiglobulin test and possibly an elution. Other tests may be affected, and transfusion of incompatible blood may be required.

Topics covered in this unit allow the technician to relate test methods and results to specific clinical conditions. It is vital to not only perform laboratory tests but also to relate those results to specific patients. The technician's role in prevention and diagnosis of clinical conditions is important and should be emphasized in the classroom and clinic.

CASE STUDY 10

A prenatal patient was seen at an obstetrical clinic for a routine visit. This was the third pregnancy for the patient. Blood tests were ordered. The test results were as follows:

Anti-A	*Anti-B*	*Anti-A,B*	*Anti-D*	*Weak D*
4+	0	4+	0	Negative

Antibody Screen: negative at all phases

1. Is there any possibility that Rh hemolytic disease of the newborn will be present in this infant?
2. Can steps be taken to prevent Rh HDN in future pregancies? If so, outline these steps in detail.
3. Would the answers to questions #1 or 2 change if the father were a known Rh negative?

CASE STUDY 11

A patient experienced fever and chills during the transfusion of a unit of packed red blood cells. The transfusion was stopped and an appropriate investigation was performed. As a result of the investigation, clerical checks revealed no discrepancies, no signs of hemolysis were present in any posttransfusion samples, and the direct antiglobulin tests were negative on all samples.

1. Is it necessary to do any further testing for this investigation? Explain.
2. Was the most likely cause of this reaction a red cell antigen and antibody reaction? Explain.
3. What probably caused this reaction? How could future reactions be prevented?

CASE STUDY 12

A 55-year-old male, previously diagnosed with hypertension, presented at his physician's office with severe anemia. The physician admitted him to the local hospital and ordered 2 units of packed red cells for transfusion. The results of the pretransfusion testing included the following:

Anti-A	*Anti-B*	*Anti-A,B*	*Anti-D*	*Weak D Test*
4+	0	4+	0	Positive

Antibody Screen: Cells I and II positive in AHG
Antibody Identification: Inconclusive, positive in all cells at AHG
DAT: 3+ with anti-IgG
All crossmatches 2+ incompatible at AHG
Medications: Aldomet (hypertensive drug)

1. What is most likely the cause of the anemia seen in this patient? What may have created the problem? How could it be corrected?
2. What is the Rh type of this patient? Explain.
3. Should this patient be transfused? Why or why not?

REVIEW QUESTIONS

1. The most common cause of hemolytic disease of the newborn is
   a. ABO antibodies
   b. anti-D
   c. anti-K
   d. none of the above
2. Rh immune globulin is administered after
   a. 12 weeks
   b. 20 weeks
   c. 28 weeks
   d. labor has begun
3. An Rh-positive infant is born to an Rh-negative mother. Rh immune globulin is administered
   a. always
   b. if the mother has no anti-D in the serum
   c. when the maternal antibody screen is positive
   d. only in cases of stillbirth
4. A fetal screen test is performed. No rosettes are seen on the microscopic examination. This test is interpreted as
   a. negative
   b. positive
   c. inconclusive
   d. improperly performed

5. A cord blood sample was evaluated. Test results were as follows:

Anti-A	*Anti-B*	*Anti-A,B*	*Anti-D*
4+	4+	4+	4+

The most likely explanation of these results is that
   a. the infant is AB positive
   b. the infant has ABO and Rh HDN
   c. the sample was not properly washed
   d. the antisera were all contaminated
6. A hemolytic transfusion reaction frequently has direct antiglobulin test results that are
   a. positive in both pretransfusion and posttransfusion samples
   b. negative in both pretransfusion and posttransfusion samples
   c. positive in the pretransfusion sample and negative in the posttransfusion sample
   d. negative in the pretransfusion sample and positive in the posttransfusion sample.
7. Hemoglobinemia is most often encountered in the sample that is collected
   a. posttransfusion following a hemolytic transfusion reaction
   b. pretransfusion for any type of anemia
   c. both pretransfusion and posttransfusion for delayed transfusion reactions
   d. after a febrile reaction has occurred
8. A Kleihauer-Betke acid elution stain is performed. When the smears are examined microscopically, they may be interpreted as:
   a. fetal cells are pale pink cells; adult cells are dark pink
   b. fetal cells are dark pink cells; adult cells are pale pink
   c. all red cells are pale pink; fetal cells have a nucleus
   d. fetal cells are seen as unstained; adult cells are pink
9. In autoimmune hemolytic anemia, the test results are
   a. direct antiglobulin and antibody screen tests always positive
   b. direct antiglobulin test always positive and antibody screen test always negative
   c. direct antiglobulin test always negative and antibody screen sometimes positive
   d. direct antiglobulin test always positive and antibody screen sometimes positive
10. In autoimmune hemolytic anemia, the autocontrol test in the antibody screen is
   a. negative
   b. positive
   c. variable
   d. not performed

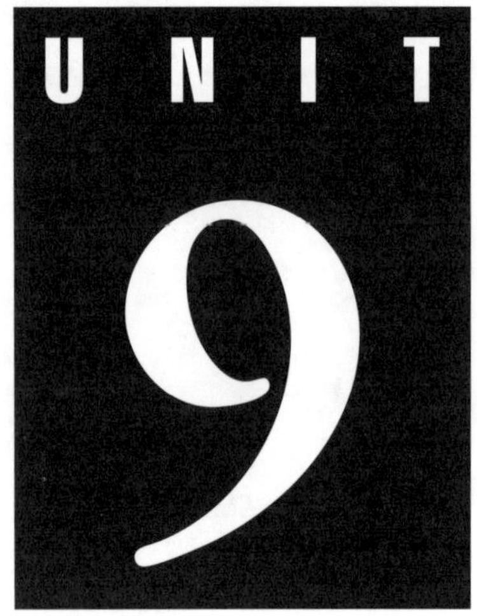

Quality Assurance in the Blood Bank

LEARNING OBJECTIVES

After studying this unit, it is the responsibility of the student to know the following objectives:

- **Define terms listed in the glossary.**
- **Describe general quality assurance in the blood bank laboratory.**
- **Differentiate quality assurance from quality control.**
- **Perform quality control on daily-use reagents.**
- **Perform temperature monitoring on blood bank equipment.**

GLOSSARY

external proficiency testing specimens for evaluation of test methods that are distributed to laboratories by an outside agency.

internal proficiency testing specimens for evaluation of test methods that originate within the laboratory.

peer review group group of peers that evaluate the performance of the laboratory.

quality assurance efforts of all personnel to monitor and evaluate all aspects of laboratory testing to improve patient care.

quality control series of procedures to monitor test systems.

INTRODUCTION

Quality assurance is important in all areas of the laboratory. **Quality control** of reagents and equipment is a small portion of the overall quality assurance system in the blood bank. Determination of quality test performance begins with the collection of specimens and terminates with the successful transfusion of blood components. Ancillary systems of the quality assurance system include quality control of blood collection and component preparation as well as **internal** and **external proficiency testing.** The overall quality control system will be briefly outlined in this unit, with emphasis on laboratory testing.

QUALITY ASSURANCE VERSUS QUALITY CONTROL

Quality assurance is a comprehensive program that strives to monitor and evaluate all aspects of test performance. A summary of components of quality assurance is found in Table 9.1.

Quality control includes the components of monitoring the testing systems. It is a narrow focus within the larger scope of quality assurance. Quality control is composed of a system to monitor test methods, reagents, instrumentation, and other items. The specific focus of this unit will be quality control within the blood bank laboratory.

SPECIMEN COLLECTION

Quality control of specimen collection may not always be under the control of the laboratory. It is, however, the technician's responsibility to determine to the best of his or her ability that the specimen is properly collected and originated from the patient that is identified on the label. The labeling criteria for individual blood samples varies by institution. Computer-generated labels may be used. All labels should include the information summarized in Table 9.2. Samples that are not properly identified should not be accepted for testing. Specimen collection manuals must be available in all patient areas for reference use of all personnel.

Table 9.1. Components of Laboratory Quality Assurance

Components
Personnel
Specimen collection and labeling
Procedures
Reagents
Quality of materials and instruments
Reporting methods
Financial components
Patient and physician satisfaction

Table 9.2. Labeling Blood Specimens for Blood Bank Tests

Patient's first and last names
Identification number
Date
Identification of the phlebotomist

The blood sample should be collected in the appropriate tube for the test being performed. Most blood bank tests are performed using a clotted sample. For the direct antiglobulin test, an EDTA sample is acceptable.

STANDARD OPERATING PROCEDURE MANUALS

A standard operating procedure (SOP) manual should be available in the blood bank laboratory. This manual summarizes procedures used in the department. Information on specimen collection, quality control, record keeping, test procedures, and emergency procedures are a few of the items that may be found in this manual. The manual must be reviewed and revised on a regular basis by administrative personnel.

REAGENT QUALITY CONTROL PROCEDURES

Quality control is performed on reagents used in test procedures. Reagents used in routine tests have quality control procedures performed daily. If multiple work shifts are employed in the institution, the control procedures are performed at the beginning of each shift.

ANTISERA CONTROLS

Controls for antisera are two separate controls, using cells that are positive and negative for the antigen detected in the test. The control method uses the standard test procedure for that antisera. For anti-A, anti-B, anti-A,B, and anti-Rh_o(D),

EXERCISE 51 SPECIMEN IDENTIFICATION

In pairs, students should:

1. Perform a venipuncture, observing all safety precautions.
2. Collect a plain red-top specimen.
3. Label the sample using the guidelines in Table 9.2.
4. Reverse roles.
5. The instructor should check the results.

the control procedure uses a 1:1 ratio of antisera and cells. Potent antisera such as anti-A and anti-B may be diluted to make certain that the antisera will detect weak antigens. Whenever possible, cells chosen as the positive control should be heterozygous. This helps to determine that the antisera will detect antigens in a state of weakened expression.

Antisera not used on a daily basis are tested when used. These antisera are also tested with positive and negative controls, using the same guidelines previously described.

QUALITY CONTROL OF ANTI-HUMAN GLOBULIN SERA

Quality control of anti-human globulin (AHG) sera is performed using cells that are coated with antibody. Combination of the AHG sera with check cells serves this purpose as the daily procedure.

QUALITY CONTROL OF CELL PRODUCTS

Quality control of cell products begins with visual examination of the supernatant. Cells that exhibit hemolysis may be considered not acceptable for use. If the hemolysis can be removed with one wash, the cells may be used on that day.

Additionally, reverse grouping cells, antibody screen cells, and check cells should be tested each day of use. Reverse grouping cells are tested with an antisera that produces a positive result and one that will not produce a positive result. Antibody screen cells are tested with a weak saline reactive antibody and a weak AHG reactive antibody. Check cells are tested with AHG sera to serve as a positive control. A negative control should also be performed using a solution that would not be expected to produce a positive result.

Cells for use with antibody identification panels do not require quality control. Visual examination and careful observation for testing discrepancies serve as acceptable quality control.

EXERCISE 52 SELECTION OF CELLS FOR USE DURING QUALITY CONTROL OF ANTISERA

In pairs or small groups, the students should obtain an antigram that accompanies an antibody identification panel. The students should choose cells that are appropriate to use as positive and negative controls for the following antisera:

Anti-C
Anti-K
Anti-Jk^a
Anti-Fy^b

RECORDS OF REAGENT QUALITY CONTROL

Records of daily reagent quality control should be made each day and maintained for review by accrediting agencies. These records should include the information summarized in Table 9.3.

All discrepancies should be recorded and corrective action taken. The corrective action should also be permanently recorded.

Table 9.3. Records of Daily Reagent Controls

Date of testing
Source of reagent used
Expiration dates
Lot numbers of reagents
Visual inspection of reagents
Identification of person performing testing

EXERCISE 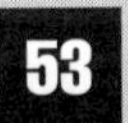

RECORD SHEET FOR REAGENT QUALITY CONTROL

Each student should prepare a record sheet for quality control. The guidelines in Table 9.3 should be used as a reference. The reagents included should be those summarized in the previous sections. This record sheet will be used for Exercise 54.

EXERCISE 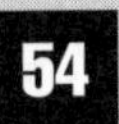

REAGENT QUALITY CONTROL EXERCISE

Each student should perform the following quality control exercise.

Equipment
Gloves
Goggles
10 × 75 or 12 × 75 mm test tubes
Transfer pipet
Test tube rack
Marking pen
0.85% saline in a wash bottle
Anti-A, anti-B, anti-A,B
Anti-D (Rh control, if required)
AHG sera
LISS (or other enhancement media)

EXERCISE 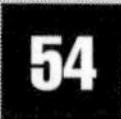 REAGENT QUALITY CONTROL EXERCISE *(continued)*

6% albumin
A and B reverse grouping cells
Antibody screen cells
Check cells
Diluted antisera for a saline reactive antibody
Diluted antisera for an AHG reactive antibody
Serological centrifuge
37°C heat block
Agglutination viewer
Record sheet from Exercise 53
Puncture-proof biohazard container

Procedure

The use of barrier protection items, including gloves and goggles, are required for this entire exercise.

ABO Antiseras

1. Label two sets of tubes for forward ABO grouping. Label 1 set "Positive" and the second "Negative."
2. Place 1 drop of the appropriate antisera into each of the six tubes.
3. Into each tube of the positive set, place one drop of cells that will produce a positive result with that antisera. For example, place 1 drop of A cells into the anti-A and anti-A,B tubes.
4. Into the negative set, add 1 drop of group O cells to each tube (screen cells may be used).
5. Centrifuge for 15 seconds. Examine using an agglutination viewer and record results. Record and correct any discrepancies noted.

Rh Antisera

1. Label two tubes for Rh typing. Label one "Positive" and the second "Negative."
2. Place 1 drop of anti-D into each tube.
3. Into the tube labeled "Positive," place 1 drop of Rh-positive cells.
4. Into the tube labeled "Negative," place 1 drop of Rh-negative cells.
5. Centrifuge for 15 to 30 seconds as designated for the type of antisera being used. Examine using an agglutination viewer and record results. Record and correct any discrepancies noted.

AHG Sera and Check Cells

1. Label two tubes "AHG." Label one "Positive" and one "Negative." Note that the positive tube serves as a positive control for both AHG and check cells.

EXERCISE 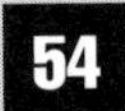 REAGENT QUALITY CONTROL EXERCISE *(continued)*

2. Label one tube "Saline." This will serve as a negative tube for check cells.
3. Place 2 drops of AHG sera into both "AHG" tubes.
4. Place 2 drops of saline into "Saline" tube.
5. Place 1 drop of check cells into the positive tube and the saline tube. Note that the positive tube serves as a positive control for the AHG sera and the check cells. The saline tube serves as a negative control for the check cells.
6. Into the negative tube place 1 drop of antibody screen cells.
7. Centrifuge for 15 seconds. Examine using an agglutination viewer and record results. Record and correct any discrepancies noted.

ABO Reverse Grouping Cells

1. Label two sets of tubes for reverse grouping. Label one set "Positive" and the second set "Negative."
2. Place 2 drops of anti-A into the A tube and 2 drops of anti-B into the B tube of the "Positive" set.
3. Into the "negative" set place 2 drops of anti-B into the A tube and 2 drops of anti-A into the B tube.
4. Place 1 drop of the appropriate reverse group cell into the correct tube.
5. Centrifuge for 15 seconds. Examine using an agglutination viewer, and record results. Record and correct any discrepancies noted.

Antibody Screen Cells

1. Label two sets of tubes for antibody screen. Label one set "positive" and the second set "negative."
2. Using an antigram for the screen cells, choose an antisera that will produce a positive result in the saline phase and will react with one of the cells. Choose a second antisera that will react with the other cell at the AHG phase. Using the positive set of tubes, place 2 drops of the appropriate antisera into the correct tube.
3. Into each tube of the "negative" set place 2 drops of 6% albumin.
4. Place 1 drop of the appropriate cell into each tube.
5. Centrifuge for 15 seconds, examine with an agglutination viewer, and record results.
6. Add 2 drops of LISS (or other enhancement media) to each tube.
7. Centrifuge for 20 seconds, examine with an agglutination viewer, and record results.
8. Incubate for 5 to 15 minutes (incubation time is dependent on the media being used) in a 37°C heat block.
9. Centrifuge for 20 seconds. Examine using an agglutination viewer and record results.

EXERCISE 

REAGENT QUALITY CONTROL EXERCISE *(continued)*

10. Wash three or four times and add 2 drops of AHG sera to each tube.
11. Centrifuge for 15 seconds and examine using an agglutination viewer. Record and correct any discrepancies noted.
12. Add 1 drop of check cells to each tube. Centrifuge, examine, and record results.
13. Interpret all results to determine discrepancies. Note all discrepancies and determine the cause.
14. Dispose of all biohazardous waste in a puncture-proof biohazard container.

EQUIPMENT QUALITY CONTROL

All equipment and instruments must have quality control procedures and preventive maintenance performed by a designated schedule. The quality control includes temperature records on any equipment that are temperature dependent. This equipment is summarized in Table 9.4.

Additional equipment maintenance includes checking the speed of centrifuges with a tachometer at least every 6 months. Checking the timers of centrifuges with a stopwatch should be done periodically. Automated cell washers require varied quality control related to the specific functions of the instrument. The operating manual should be consulted for these specific requirements.

EXTERNAL QUALITY ASSURANCE

The procedures outlined in the previous sections describe the internal quality control in the blood bank laboratory. External quality assurance is provided from outside agencies. The Food and Drug Administration and some state agencies issue licenses that permit the laboratories to operate.

Table 9.4. Equipment Requiring Temperature Records

Heat blocks
Water baths
Refrigerators
Freezers
Refrigerated centrifuges
Rh viewing boxes
Platelet incubators

External proficiency testing is provided by **peer review groups** such as the College of American Pathologists (CAP) and American Association of Blood Banks (AABB). These agencies provide voluntary review of blood banks. Some of these, such as the CAP, also periodically provide samples for analysis. These samples include tests that are routinely performed in the blood bank, such as ABO, Rh, antibody screen, and identification and direct antiglobulin test. The results of these analyses are then assessed by the CAP and a report is sent to the laboratory.

SUMMARY

Quality assurance is a broad concept that monitors all aspects of testing. Quality control is a part of the quality assurance system that includes a set of procedures performed daily or on an established schedule. Quality control procedures require that most reagents be tested on the day of use to determine that achieved results will be accurate. Quality control of equipment must be performed to determine that the temperatures and basic functions are appropriate for the tests being performed. Results of these procedures must be recorded and maintained.

External agencies provide either mandatory or voluntary review to ascertain that operations follow established practices. Some of the voluntary agencies also provide test samples to be analyzed.

All aspects of quality assurance and quality control are important in providing appropriate patient care. Following the established procedures will aid in determining that test procedures, reagents, and equipment are as accurate and appropriate as possible.

REVIEW QUESTIONS

1. Quality control for antibody screen cells consists of testing with
   a. weak anti-A,B
   b. 6% albumin
   c. anti-human globulin antibody
   d. check cells
2. Daily quality control does *not* include
   a. temperature monitoring
   b. controls for antibody screen cells
   c. examination of fluid on cell products
   d. external proficiency testing
3. Cells in antibody identification panels require quality control testing
   a. daily regardless of use
   b. on the day of use
   c. with each use
   d. at no time

4. Corrective steps taken for discrepancies found in daily quality control
   a. are not important
   b. must be recorded
   c. do not require documentation
   d. follow specific guidelines
5. Specimen collection requires proper labeling. The item that is *not* required on the label is
   a. patient's name
   b. identification number
   c. anticoagulant
   d. date
6. Quality control of centrifuges includes
   a. measurement of saline volume
   b. balance check
   c. examination of supernatant fluid
   d. check of timer accuracy
7. Controls of antisera not used on a daily basis are performed
   a. daily
   b. monthly
   c. when used
   d. at no time
8. A positive control for anti-D would consist of
   a. group O cells
   b. Rh-positive cells
   c. Rh-negative cells
   d. heterozygous C cells
9. Anti-human globulin sera and check cells are combined to form a positive control for
   a. only AHG sera
   b. only check cells
   c. both AHG sera and check cells
   d. neither AHG sera nor check cells
10. ABO reagents used for forward and reverse grouping have quality control assessment
    a. daily
    b. weekly
    c. monthly
    d. at no time

APPENDIX A • ANSWERS TO REVIEW QUESTIONS AND CASE STUDIES

UNIT 1

1. a
2. b
3. b
4. a
5. c
6. c
7. c
8. d
9. a
10. b

UNIT 2

1. c
2. d
3. d
4. e
5. a
6. a
7. c
8. a
9. d
10. d
11. b
12. c
13. d

UNIT 3

1. c
2. d
3. b
4. b
5. d
6. d
7. a
8. b
9. c
10. b

CASE STUDY 1

1. Group A; based on forward grouping.
2. Forward and reverse groups do not match.
3. Do not usually perform reverse group on a newborn because they do not have their own antibodies.
4. Knowing the mother's blood group explains the antibodies present in the serum.

CASE STUDY 2

1. Subgroup of A, with anti-A_1 in serum.
2. Forward and reverse groups do not match. Forward group appears as a group A. Reverse group appears as a group O.
3. Anti-A_1 antibody is stimulated by exposure to A_1 antigen.
4. No errors have occurred in testing. The results can be explained. The patient presents as a subgroup of A with an anti-A_1.

UNIT 4

1. a
2. c
3. a
4. b
5. c
6. d
7. b
8. c
9. c
10. b

CASE STUDY 3

1. Rh typing is invalid because the control is positive.
2. An autoantibody or increased plasma protein.
3. Repeat Rh type with saline antisera.
4. O negative.

CASE STUDY 4

1. Weak D positive because it occurred after anti-human globulin.
2. Rh positive as a donor because he has the D antigen.
3. Rh negative blood is administered for transfusion so that she does not receive an antigen that she does not possess.
4. No further tests necessary.

UNIT 5

1. b
2. d
3. d
4. b
5. d
6. a
7. c
8. c
9. b
10. b

UNIT 6

1. c
2. b
3. c
4. c
5. c
6. b
7. d
8. c
9. a
10. a

CASE STUDY 5

1. Anti-Jk^a.
2. Enzymes would enhance Anti-Jk^a.
3. Negative for the Jk^a antigen.
4. Antigen type donor's cells for the Jk^a antigen; only antigen negative cells should be transfused.

CASE STUDY 6

1. Direct antiglobulin test; use polyspecific and monospecific anti-human globulin (AHG) sera to determine the exact etiology of the antibody.
2. Elution to remove antibody from cells so that the antibody can be identified.
3. A panel on the serum is not necessary because no antibody is detected in the serum.

UNIT 7

1. c	6. a
2. a	7. a
3. c	8. b
4. b	9. d
5. c	10. b

CASE STUDY 7

1. O negative.
2. ABO group, Rh type, antibody screen, and crossmatch of all units.
3. Complete crossmatch procedure will need to be completed to determine compatibility, even if the units have been completely transfused.

CASE STUDY 8

1. Yes, the patient needs therapy with red cells, platelets, and possibly white blood cells.
2. Sensitivity to white blood cells needs to be considered so that the patient will not experience a reaction to any white blood cells in a unit of packed red cells. This is a factor that is important for the patient's comfort and safety. This patient should be transfused with units of red cells that are considered to be leukocyte poor.
3. If the white blood cell count is extremely low, transfusions of leukocyte concentrate may be considered to help to fight the unresponsive infection.
4. The diminished platelet count is significant and may require transfusion of platelets to prevent hemorrhage.

CASE STUDY 9

1. The technician may be permitted to inform the donor that he/she is not eligible to donate blood due to the positive test for hepatitis. This fact should, however, be confirmed on donor records before deferring the donor.
2. If the donor has a positive test for hepatitis B, the blood may not be used for transfusion since it may be capable of transmitting the hepatitis B virus to a recipient.
3. When applying the labels to the unit, the technician should always discard all unused labels to prevent a clerical error.

UNIT 8

1. a
2. c
3. b
4. a
5. a
6. d
7. a
8. b
9. d
10. b

CASE STUDY 10

1. It is not likely since the mother has no anti-D in her serum.
2. Yes, Rh immune globulin may be administered antenatally and postpartum.
3. Yes, the Rh immune globulin would not need to be administered.

CASE STUDY 11

1. No, because there are no indications of hemolytic transfusion reaction.
2. No, because there are no indications of an antibody-antigen interaction.
3. Probably a reaction with an antibody to a white cell or platelet antigen. Future reactions can be prevented by providing cell products that are leukocyte poor.

CASE STUDY 12

1. Drug-induced autoimmune hemolytic anemia. Aldomet probably caused the problem. It may be corrected by removing the drug from the patient's treatment.
2. Rh type is not able to be determined. Rh-negative blood should be administered.
3. It should be avoided if possible since providing more red cells may cause more hemolysis and hence more problems.

UNIT 9

1. c
2. d
3. d
4. b
5. c
6. a
7. c
8. b
9. c
10. a

REFERENCES

Harmening, D. *Modern Blood Banking and Transfusion Practices*, ed. 3, Philadelphia: F.A. Davis, 1994.

Marshall, J. *Fundamental Skills for the Clinical Laboratory Professional.* Albany, N.Y.: Delmar, 1993.

Standards for Blood Banks and Transfusion Services, ed. 16, Arlington, Va.: American Association of Blood Banks, 1995.

Turgeon, M.L. *Fundamentals of Immunohematology*, ed. 2, Baltimore: Williams and Wilkins, 1995.

Walker, R., editor. *American Association of Blood Banks Technical Manual*, ed. 11, Arlington, Va.: American Association of Blood Banks, 1993.

Walters, N.J., Estridge, B.H., and Reynolds, A.P. *Basic Medical Laboratory Techniques.* Albany, N.Y.: Delmar, 1990.

INDEX